M000030936

the nashville diet

the nashville diet

THE 3-STEP PLAN TO
LOSE WEIGHT,
"NUTRAPLENISH" YOUR BODY,
AND ACHIEVE VIBRANT HEALTH

Marilyn Tucker, D.Ph.

LifeLine
Press

Copyright © 2003 by Marilyn Tucker

All rights reserved. No part of this publication may be reproduced or transmitted in any form or by any means electronic or mechanical, including photocopy, recording, or any information storage and retrieval system now known or to be invented, without permission in writing from the publisher, except by a reviewer who wishes to quote brief passages in connection with a review written for inclusion in a magazine, newspaper, or broadcast.

Library of Congress Cataloging-in-Publication Data on file. Available upon request
ISBN 0-89526-118-9

Published in the United States by
LifeLine Press
A Regnery Publishing Company
One Massachusetts Avenue, N.W.
Washington, DC 20001

Visit us at www.lifelinepress.com

Distributed to the trade by
National Book Network
4720-A Boston Way
Lanham, MD 20706

Printed on acid-free paper

Manufactured in the United States of America

10 9 8 7 6 5 4 3 2 1

Books are available in quantity for promotional or premium use. Write to Director of Special Sales, Regnery Publishing, Inc., One Massachusetts Avenue, N.W., Washington, DC 20001, for information on discounts and terms or call (202) 216-0600.

The information contained in this book is not a substitute for medical counseling and care. All matters pertaining to your physical health should be supervised by a health care professional.

DEDICATION

I would like to dedicate this work to the Lord and my darling daughter, Clair Brooke Chaddick. To the Lord for giving me my health, my daughter, and the privilege of giving this gift of health to others. To my daughter for being with me through it all.

HOSEA 4:6.

contents

acknowledgment

many thanks to all those people who have been with me along this journey, specifically: Karen Anderson, Rhonda Adkins, Judy Burt, Daniel Bates, Barbara Baydoun, Kimberly Bender, Jay Bowden, Paula Bowden, Lynda Brown, Leanne Bush, Leslie Burbridge, Kim Camp, Julie Chambers, Melissa Cureton, George Cocchini, Joe Cocchini, Ann Ewers, Cameron Gaither, Heather Gaither, Kelly Garrett, Susan Houston, Christopher Huffman, Erma Jackson, Patricia Jackson, Wayne Jackson, Deb Joysey, LifeLine Press, Sue Martin, Bill McVey, Jerry Nelson, Joel Pettegrew, Mac Ross, Marji Ross, Kim Shoun, Mike Shoun, Melody Smiley, Mike Smiley, Joan Stadler, Mick Stadler, Jim Stein, Heather Stevens, Lisa Stickle, Eugene Tucker, Jim Ward, and "Ernie the Attorney" Williams.

My thanks also to all my clients, for their dedication and courage to walk the path.

introduction

in september of 1993 I left my busy business for what was supposed to be a ninety-day leave of absence for the express purpose of getting well. I'd been sick for several years, gradually getting worse until I'd reached the point where working became very difficult for me. I was exhausted all the time, in a continuous mental fog, and my joints and muscles ached constantly, as though I had the flu. ItC was time for me to forget everything else and focus on putting an end to this thing. "I'm a pharmacist," I thought, "I ought to be able to figure a way out." So I went home for ninety days.

Five years passed before I came back out.

Early in 1998 I dragged myself out of bed to visit my doctor's office, where I listened to this most dedicated of physicians tell me there was no more he could do for me. He'd sent me to more than a dozen specialists, none of whom could alleviate my fibromyalgia, my chronic fatigue syndrome, and my soaring weight. I'd been on antibiotics for five years straight, alternating them in a futile effort to fend off recurring bronchial pneumonia and sinus infections. I'd taken antiviral and antifungal medications, as well as pills for low thyroid. My immune system had pretty much crashed, and now I was being told there was nothing to be done about it. I cried, went home, got back into bed, and cried some more. I knew I couldn't live like this anymore. I prayed for the Lord to either heal me or take me, and I began to prepare for Him to choose the second option. Then the phone rang.

The person on the phone was the father of the little boy my daughter was tutoring, making yet another effort to get me to try something called nutraceuticals. His wife had been telling me about this class of completely natural supplements for quite a while, and I'd been rebuffing her politely. I wasn't interested.

As a pharmacist trained in the realm of chemicals, I was skeptical about meaningful health benefits coming from capsules with ground-up plant matter in them, which is basically what nutraceuticals are. The general idea of alternative treatments held some interest for me. For me, acceptable "alternative medicine" consisted of 10,000 daily milligrams of ascorbic acid, another chemical which I assumed was actually vitamin C (mistakenly, I later learned). For the most part, my mind was closed to true alternative medicine. At the time, I considered it lunatic fringe stuff.

This man on the phone was no lunatic-fringer, however, and I agreed to let him send me some informational material, which I didn't read. He followed up by sending me a few weeks' supply of the nutraceutical products he thought I should try, which I promptly put aside without even opening the bottles.

But the gentleman called me one last time to see if I'd started taking the capsules. As I started to tell him how much I knew already—me being a pharmacist, and all—he interrupted me and said, "Oh yes, I can see what you're doing is working *real well.*"

That got me. I knew he was right. I had reached the end of my options. I promised him I'd take the capsules daily for three weeks. In total desperation, I finally began swallowing the nutraceuticals.

I felt the difference immediately. The mental fog began to lift in a day or two. The exhaustion that had defined my existence for so long showed the first hint of improvement. My previously nonstop food cravings eased up a tad. After more than half a decade of wanting to do nothing but lie in bed and eat, I found myself wanting to get out of bed and do something besides eat. Within three weeks I was able to do twenty-five minutes on a StairMaster—an exhilarating achievement for somebody who had trouble walking around the house just three weeks earlier. I was on my way back!

Since then, the program I developed to help myself to lose weight and overcome illness has evolved into the Nashville Diet. It's what allowed me to completely recover what I've come to call my vibrant health. It's why I now wear a size 2. It's why I have more strength and lean muscle mass, not to mention less cellulite, than most high school girls. It's why my body fat has dropped from 38 percent to 14 percent, my cholesterol count from 287 to 145, and my triglyceride count from nearly 300 to 85. It's why I no longer crave sweets or have any interest at all in chocolate.

Many people tell me I look ten to fifteen years younger than I did five years ago. For a long time people who knew me well literally did not recognize me if they hadn't seen me recently. My energy, once missing in action, is now high enough to run a demanding but rewarding business, work fifteen hours a day, and win ballroom dancing competitions in my spare time.

My journey from there to here—from fat to lean, from bedridden to bursting with health and energy—is what inspired me to write about my health and diet discoveries. The book, however, is not about me. It's about you. It exists to show you how to make the same transition I did. I wrote it to provide you with precisely the information you need to shed the debilitating fat that's been burdening you for so long.

The first thing I did with my returning mental clarity and recovering body was research those nutraceutical capsules that had turned my life around. The combination of nutraceuticals I took was a rudimentary (and much weaker) version of the nutritional supplement regimen that forms the basis of the Nashville Diet you'll be following. Taking advantage of my pharmacy training, I was able to tweak my supplementation early on to speed my recovery and lose fat more efficiently. More importantly, I was able for the first time to discover the "why" of my health and weight problems, and the "how" of the nutraceuticals' ability to solve those problems.

This knowledge led me to discover and capitalize on the groundbreaking principals I now use in the Nashville Diet and at my clinic.

I'm living proof that those principals hold the key to health and weight loss. You'll be learning about these principals and how to apply them so you can achieve the lean, healthy, energetic body that's rightfully yours.

You are overweight because you are undernourished. As counterintuitive as it sounds, this is the bedrock truth of the Nashville Diet. This simple fact was a stunning eye-opener for me, one of those revelations that are hard to believe at first but turns out to make so much sense you wonder why the whole world isn't aware of it. The Nashville Diet will show you how to get nourished so that fat loss will follow.

Nutraceuticals feed you in ways food no longer can. The capsules that got me out of bed and into a size 2 aren't miracle drugs. In fact, they're not drugs at all. They don't "cure" your health problems. They're not "diet pills." They simply provide the nutrients your body needs to resist disease, function properly, and process food efficiently enough to eliminate the cravings that make you fat. The Nashville Diet works because it describes the precise combination of nutrients you need to restore your internal health and lose fat—and delivers them in the form of nutraceuticals. Just why food itself doesn't get the job done is another story that awaits you in the pages ahead.

Your overall health and your body fat levels cannot be separated. It makes no sense to try to shed excess fat in order to be healthier, though most diets urge you to do exactly that. You must instead improve your internal health in order to shed that excess fat. Nothing else will work for long, as thousands of fad diets have proven over the years. That's why the Nashville Diet focuses equally on losing fat and gaining health.

We live in a toxic world, and it's keeping us fat. Anybody not holed up in a cave is all too aware that we're constantly taking in poison from the air we breathe, the food we eat, the water we drink, and the countless synthetic chemicals that we've chosen to share the earth with. Yet the connection between accumulated toxicity in your body and the difficulty we have letting go of fat is never emphasized and seldom recognized in any commercial diet. The Nashville Diet will teach you how to help your body shed fat by ridding it of long-stored toxins and keeping new ones out.

Quick weight loss makes you fat. Absolutely the worst way in the world to lose weight is to force yourself to eat less than you want to. Yet virtually every get-thin-quick scheme asks you to do precisely that, one way or another. For reasons you'll be learning about, the only progress you'll make with get-thin-quick tricks is toward a higher weight than you started with. The Nashville Diet doesn't pay much attention to "dieting" in the usual sense of the word, because the only way to get lean and stay that way is to eliminate the imbalances that make you want to eat too much in the first place.

On Valentine's Day, 1999, I started accepting clients at my new Vibrant Health Systems clinic. Today, the clinic has become something of an institution in Nashville, a place where people from all walks of life leave fad diets and get-thin-quick schemes behind and get down to the real business of becoming permanently lean and fit by reclaiming their vibrant health. I am a woman twice blessed—first for being allowed to come back from the brink, and then for being given the rewarding life of playing a part in so many people's changed lives.

In the pages that follow, you'll find the same program you'd get if you enrolled in my Nashville clinic. The book is divided into three parts that correspond with the three co-equal components of the Nashville Diet. Part One describes the central problem that underlies your weight problems—undernourished cells resulting from the nutrient-depleted food we've been living with for several decades (not coincidentally, the same several decades that ushered in the current obesity crisis). You'll then learn about the solution to that problem, a nutraceutical-based supplementation program I call nutraplenishing. Part Two explains another important and often ignored factor in your weight problems—toxin buildup in your bodily systems. It also provides you with a lot of different ways to reduce your toxic overload, thereby encouraging fat loss. Part Three is the actual diet section of the program, but it contains none of the typical advice found in typical failure-prone diets. The strategy that works has you choosing healthy, natural "live" versions of the foods you already enjoy. You'll learn how to make that simple and satisfying transition, and why it leads so successfully to weight loss.

There are two things you won't find in this book, however. One is an overload of technical information. I have purposefully left out detailed discussions of the science underlying each aspect of the program for a very good reason—you don't need it. I do encourage you (as I encourage all my clients) to go out and get more information about all the topics we deal with in this book. Knowledge is power, and the more you know about how your body works and what's in the food you give it the more control you'll have over your weight, your health and your life.

But the emphasis of this book is on action, not theory. My intention is to give you a program you can use to take care of your health and body fat issues once and for all. I've done the research for you. Your job is to put it to work for your own benefit.

The other thing you won't find in this book is the standard promise to lose a certain number of pounds in a certain number of days. First of all, everybody's different, so everybody loses fat at his or her own pace. Also, for reasons that will become clear as you progress through the book, "losing pounds" isn't what fat-to-lean is all about. Most important of all, such a claim reflects the old, discredited way of thinking about health and body weight. If you're looking for the lastest miracle diet, you won't find it here. But if you've had it with yo-yo dieting and are ready to get healthy and lean for life, you've come to the right place!

I can't predict how long it will take you to get all the way from fat to lean. But I do know that if you stick with me on this program you *will* get there. And because the Nashville Diet gets you healthy as well as trim, you'll stay that way for the rest of your life.

1

NUTRAPLENISH YOUR BODY

| 1 |

THE PROBLEM:
nutrient depletion

the first thing you need to know is the most important thing I'm ever going to tell you:

It's not your fault.

It's not your fault that you've been fighting a losing battle for as long as you can remember against those ten, twenty, or thirty extra pounds, or maybe even more.

It's not your fault that you've tested your willpower against any number of deprivation diets—only to learn all too soon that unchecked cravings are stronger than willpower.

It's not your fault that you've ridden the weight roller coaster for all these years, getting a little taste of what a leaner body feels like before shooting up again to your former high weight, or beyond.

It's not you're fault if you're too often irritable, listless, miserable. Gosh, who wouldn't be?

It's not your fault that you feel terrible about your situation—frustrated, desperate, even defeated.

None of it is your fault because the state of food and nutrition in our country today virtually guarantees that you'll be overweight. In fact, your desire to consume extra calories is actually a natural response to nutritional reality. And since none of the so-called solutions address that reality, they do nothing to solve the problem.

That's all about to change for you.

YOU'RE NOT ALONE

The second thing I want you to know is that you're not alone.

You're probably already familiar with the sad statistics. They tell us that three out of four Americans are overweight and one in three are actually obese. If you want to confirm those statistics, just go outside and look around.

I'm not just talking about numbers, though. Yes, you are by no means the only person struggling with being overweight. But more important, you're not the only one struggling with the misery and sense of hopelessness that goes with it.

I see this all the time. Almost every new client breaks down and cries on her first day. They come to me after years of accumulated frustration. They're burdened with self-doubt and guilt. More often than not, they're desperate. And when they see that their condition is not the result of any weakness on their part, and that so many other women and men are (or were) in the same boat . . . well, let's just say it's a very emotional moment. It's an emotion I have felt myself, and I understand it deeply.

So when I tell you you're not alone, I mean it in a personal way. I've been where you are. I want to help you. And I'm going to stay with you every step of the way until you're where I am now—healthy, lean, vibrant, and happy.

THERE'S HOPE

I want you to know one more thing: There is hope. You can get rid of the extra fat, revive the Vibrant Health that is your birthright, and start living a life of energy, achievement, and joy.

You can do all that because unlike any other weight-loss or diet program, the one I'm offering you deals directly with the true problem. And what might that true problem be, you ask? In a nutshell, it is this:

You, like most Americans, are undernourished.

Does that surprise you? Do you feel undernourished? Sure, you feel tired and weak, and you carry around a huge appetite and have constant cravings. But undernourished? *How can you be undernourished and overfed at the same time?*

Easily. And I'm going to show you how and why.

You'll see that being undernourished is the reason for your ongoing food cravings. And you're going to take care of those cravings permanently.

I am going to show you how to thoroughly nourish every cell in your body so you will no longer have any desire to eat more than you should. You'll do it with the aid of some of the most powerful natural nutrition providers ever known to humankind.

You're also going to understand that we live on a toxic planet. And you're going to take steps to rid your body of the health-threatening, fat-feeding toxins that such a planet inflicts upon you.

Most of all, you're going to change how you think about nutrition. You'll still enjoy eating. But probably for the first time in your life, your focus will be on providing your body with the nutrition it needs rather than the food it doesn't need.

You're going to solve your weight problem once and for all. You're going to step off the diet roller coaster and be healthy. You're going to reclaim your life, your body, and your health.

I see people do it every day on my system. I did it myself. And there's no doubt in my mind that you'll do it too.

OVERFED AND UNDERNOURISHED

I cringe whenever I hear this phrase:

"Dr. Marilyn, I promise I'm going to eat right from now on."

I know the person means well. I know she wants to get lean and healthy, and that she's been told all her life that "eating right" is the way to do it. And I know her vow was probably occasioned by leftover guilt from the whipped-cream casserole she craved and ate the night before.

But as patient a person as I am, I feel like screaming every time some-body tells me he or she is going to "eat right." I always manage to resist the urge to scream. But I do give an honest response that's not at all what they expect to hear: "You can't."

It is virtually impossible today to "eat right." You just can't do it.

Why not? Because our food has lost its nutritive qualities. It's pretty close to empty. In fact, most of the food you use in the kitchen to prepare your meals has little more to offer nutritionally than that whipped-cream casserole.

To put it another way, our food is depleted of the natural nutrients that our cells need to function.

As human beings we consume food to provide our body with protein, carbohydrates, and fats. Those we get, though too often the wrong kind, in the wrong amounts, and laced with contaminants.

We also eat to feed our cells vital natural plant substances known as phytochemicals, as well as vitamins, minerals, enzymes, and probiotics (good microbes). But the unavoidable reality is that today's food supply doesn't deliver the goods. And because of that, you're undernourished no matter what you eat.

That's the crux of the problem. It's what leads to excess body fat (for reasons I'll explain soon). The only way to go from fat to lean is to com-pensate for this depletion.

None of the diet and nutrition advice out there even attempts to do that. The standard approach to weight loss tells you to eat this, to not eat that, to consume this much at that time, to exercise for a certain length of time, etc. That's all well and good; we'll be doing that here too. But as long as you're not getting any real nutrition, none of that's going to matter. Nutrition is absolutely fundamental for any eating plan. Without the nutrients you need, nothing will work.

But I'll say it again. You can't get those nutrients from food anymore. It's just not going to happen.

WHAT WENT WRONG

There are several reasons for our impoverished food supply:

- *Soil depletion.* Farming practices have robbed the soil of the chemical compounds that plants convert to nutrients.
- *Fertilizers.* The synthetic chemicals force-fed to the land add insufficient and incorrect minerals that further weaken the soil.
- *"Green harvesting."* For commercial reasons, fruits and vegetables are picked before the nutrients have had a chance to form.
- *Time.* Shipping, storage, shelf-life, and home storage diminish whatever nutrients are left.
- *Processing.* Milling, freezing, preserving and canning eliminate nutrients.
- *Preparation.* Washing, peeling, and cooking further drain food of nutrients.

The most important of these factors are the first three—soil depletion, fertilizers, and green harvesting. It's worth taking a closer look at them to get an idea of what you're up against. Know your enemy!

THE CRIPPLING OF THE AMERICAN SOIL

Adam and Eve never worried about nutrients. The Garden of Eden was blessed with an abundance of nutrient-rich fruits and vegetables. All food was natural. All food was nourishing—vine-ripened and eaten as soon as it was picked, plucked, or gathered. The first couple didn't have to fight excess body fat, or hate themselves after eating a candy bar. They truly were in Paradise.

For the most part, their descendants were equally blessed. Even as they added hunting and gathering to agriculture, the fruits of their labor continued to provide real nutrition.

But things took a turn for the worse in the twentieth century. To see why, let's take a look at a fruit that Adam and Eve eventually had some experience with — the apple.

Picture a beautiful apple orchard in the rolling hills of Georgia or Washington state. This is supposed to be a source of nutrients to sustain human life — not just vitamin A and fiber but also enzymes and hundreds of phytochemicals, including compounds called flavonoids and catechins that play important roles in life-sustaining cellular chemical reactions. They all work together, making two plus two add up to six.

But those nutrients aren't created out of thin air. The only place the tree can get the raw materials to make its apples and the nutrients in them is the soil. Those materials are drawn up through the roots of the tree to the branches and eventually to the fruit. Energy from the sun is used to weave those soil elements into a tapestry of nutritional components. That's the photosynthesis you remember learning about in grade school.

Obviously, if the raw materials are scarce or missing from the soil itself, the apples' nutrients will be compromised. And, sad to report, that is precisely the status of our soil today. Modern agricultural methods, designed to meet the needs of the ever-expanding masses, have depleted the soil of nutrient-building potential. The price we've paid for a larger food supply is a nutrient-depleted food supply. Almost 100 percent of American farm soil today is generally devoid of minerals and other essentials. As a result, the foods we eat don't provide the nutrients that are vital to our health.

WHATEVER HAPPENED TO CROP ROTATION?

Soil depletion began to reach critical proportions in the 1950s when the time-honored practice of crop rotation was more or less abandoned. Crop rotation preserves the soil by changing what's planted on a certain field from year to year in a planned sequence. Because different crops extract and deposit different materials from the ground, rotating them allows the soil to replenish itself.

For example, lima beans take copper from the soil but end up returning iron to the soil by the end of the growing cycle. Corn uses that iron while removing nitrogen, but then any of a number of legumes can replace that nitrogen the next year while extracting other nutrients. And on it goes. Farmers had learned to plan their crop rotation intelligently so that the soil would be continually replenished in a harmonious, life-sustaining cycle.

The idea is at least as old as the Old Testament. It is an ancient Jewish custom to rotate crops, with a Sabbath year of rest when nothing at all is to be planted in that field. We stayed pretty close to that wise tradition until the 1950s.

Then, as the population grew, cost efficiency assumed increased importance and it became common not to rotate crops. A certain percentage of farmers still do implement a limited crop-rotation system by alternating just two crops on any given field. That's not enough. One year of drought will start a depletion cycle if only two crops are rotated. Variety is the key. The more variety, the better the soil.

Sadly, the notion of variety has faded, and you won't find very many large agricultural operations rotating more than two crops on any piece of land. Our abandonment of proper crop rotation has crippled our soils, which in turn cripples the foods that are produced in that soil.

Here's a single but revealing illustration of what this cycle has done to our food. I've found research estimating that a bowl of spinach just after World War II contained 147 milligrams of iron. According to a Department of Agriculture study, the same bowl of spinach in 1976 had just 2 milligrams of iron in it. If you assume that the iron content in spinach hasn't decreased even more since 1976 (which you shouldn't), you would have to eat more than seventy bowls of spinach

today to get the amount of nutrition you would have had in the early
'50s.

WHAT CHEMICAL FERTILIZERS HAVE WROUGHT

Why did American agriculture believe it was possible to do away with crop
rotation without sacrificing the nutritional value of the grains, vegetables,
and legumes? Because they believed that advances in the effectiveness of
fertilizers would pick up the slack. Why bother with costly crop rotation
when you can renourish the soil each year by spreading synthetic chemicals over it?

But commercial growers use synthetic fertilizers mainly to supply nitrogen, phosphorus, and potassium. They don't come close to restoring
the full delicate balance of multiple soil nutrients that nature put there.
They don't even try. The way crops were rotated would literally restore
hundreds of different vital nutrients. Now, we restore just three or four,
not coincidentally the ones that make the crops grow big and plentiful.
No thought has been given to the real nutrient value of the crops.

What's more, the fertilizers themselves rob the crops of their nutrients
by introducing nitrogen, phosphorus, and potassium in chemical forms
different from what's supposed to be in the soil. Sure, that enhances yield,
but at the cost of nutritional quality.

Using synthetic fertilizers instead of preserving the soil represents exactly the kind of quick-fix mentality that's created the modern nutritional
desert and burdened so many innocent victims with unwanted body fat
and poor health. The truth of the matter is that our cells couldn't care less
about high yield and cost efficiency in the agriculture industry. They're
much more interested in their need for old-fashioned natural nutrition.
Synthetic chemicals fed to the foods we eat are recognized by our bodies
as what they are — toxins. They're woefully inadequate as nutrients, but
they're very effective as long-term poisons in the human body.

What it comes down to is that we haven't done a good job of preserving the soil of our land. Consider this: When Columbus reached the

New World, there was, on average, a twelve-foot topsoil layer across the United States. Most of it's gone. Where I live in Tennessee, I doubt there's twelve inches of topsoil. And what there is doesn't have much to offer.

We're paying for our abuse of the soil with poor nutrition.

THE TRUE COLOR OF GREEN HARVESTING

Let's get back to our beautiful apple orchard. Why aren't those apples full of the nutrients they once used to give us? Surely we can't just blame a lack of crop rotation in this case. After all, you can't rotate fruit trees every year.

Actually, that orchard's soil is probably weak anyway. We've simply done too much intense growing for too many centuries to expect the soil to maintain its richness.

Also, keep in mind that these apples, like many other fruits, may have had the nutrition bred right out of them. Over the decades, those in commercial agriculture have bred their crops to emphasize such things as size, appearance, and yield. Nutrition's the last thing on their minds, and it's often sacrificed as they breed toward other goals.

But something else is going on with apples, and with lots of other "fresh" produce. It's sometimes called "green harvesting." That may not sound like a bad thing. In fact, I've heard the phrase "green harvesting" used to describe environmentally friendly, or sustainable, farming methods. But here I'm using it as a term synonymous with "early harvesting" or, better yet, "premature harvesting." It's another insidious modern agricultural practice responsible for our nutritional nightmare.

Simply put, most apples are harvested anywhere from two to six weeks before they're ripe—that is, while they're still green. This is a strategy designed for the purpose of shipping more apples to more places. It's also a fail-safe way to ensure that the nutrients our bodies expect from an apple won't be there.

A mature, vine-ripened apple achieves its highest nutrient load just as it's being picked. It is in the last seventy-two hours on the tree when

80 percent of the nutrients are formed, including the powerful antioxidants that are so vital to cell health. It's like a light switch is turned on seventy-two hours before full maturity and the little elves go to work making all the phytonutrients. The elves (actually photosynthetic processes) that create these last-minute nutrients also turn the apple a brighter red, give it shine, load it with juice, make it taste sweet, and give it that perfect texture—firm but easy to bite into. None of that has a chance to happen anymore.

What's more, we've been getting our food supply from depleted soil and green-harvested plants for so long that the very seeds that start the process are also depleted. It's truly a vicious circle.

IMPOSTERS IN THE PRODUCE AISLE

How do you like your red apples? Bright red, sweet, shiny, crisp, and juicy, of course—exactly what mature, nutrient-rich apples are supposed to be. That's no coincidence. Our senses have evolved in harmony with our cells' nutritional needs. We're naturally attracted to the taste, sight, smell, and feel of nourishing foods, just as we're repulsed by rotting or toxic foods.

Now, that may lead you to wonder just how serious the green-harvesting problem really is. After all, apples today may not seem all that bad. They taste okay—not great, but okay—especially if you're under forty and have no memory of what truly nutritious apples used to taste like. They're more or less red, though "bright" may be too strong an adjective. They're also sweet (sometimes), shiny (sort of), crisp (relatively speaking), and juicy (except when they're not).

True enough. But today's depleted apples are passable impostors only because there are plenty of quick-fix tricks to take care of the superficial problems caused by picking the apples before their time. For example, a green-harvested apple gets gassed, usually with nitrous oxides, soon after it's off the tree. This pressurized-gas treatment helps soften up the rock-hard immature apples.

They're also dyed red and waxed to a shine. Wonderful, isn't it? What Mother Nature accomplishes so slowly—and perfectly—modern synthetics can take care of in a few minutes. And all that's lost in the process are the nutrients that give us life and health.

For a learning moment, try slicing open one of your red supermarket apples. Check around the underside of the skin. If you see a greenish rim, you know it's been dyed on the outside. That green is closer to the color that the apple was when picked than the phony red on the outside.

That's green harvesting. Along with farming in depleted soil, it's what turns our fruit into a poor representation of genuine food. What you end up eating isn't much more than raw fiber infused with sparsely sugared water, along with some toxic chemicals from the fertilizers and pesticides for good measure.

SHIPPED, STORED, PROCESSED, AND PACKAGED

That picturesque apple orchard we've been examining may be soaked in rustic charm, but it's also soaked in toxic chemicals. Our poor, empty apples are sprayed with pesticides at every step of the process—on the tree, off the tree, as they're shipped, at market, and even in their bins along the produce aisle.

Those toxic chemicals add insult to injury. They further weaken our systems that have already been weakened by a lack of nutrients. But I won't get into the toxification of our foods in much depth here, for two reasons. One is that we'll be talking about it a lot in Part Two of this book, where I'll be showing you how to promote fat loss and feel better by detoxifying your system.

The other reason I'm holding off is to spare you too much bad news all at once. I always lose 10 pounds when I intensify my research about our food supply. The more you're aware of what's in (and not in) the food you eat, the less you'll want to eat it. Trust me, though, the good news—the solution—is coming up in the next chapter.

But let's get back to the grocery store for a little bit.

THE LONG AND WINDING ROAD

Even if you get your hands on a vine-ripened tomato grown in nutrient-rich soil (which few people ever will), it probably lost most of its nutrients long ago. The nutrients start to leech out the minute anything is picked, and by seventy-two hours after harvest, most of the few nutrients that were present at the time of picking are almost gone. And unless you grow your own fruits and vegetables or buy them at a local farmer's market, a heck of a lot more than seventy-two hours has elapsed by the time you take a bite.

Modern refrigerated transportation is definitely a plus, helping to preserve any nutrients that survived soil depletion, synthetic fertilizers, and green harvesting. But it's not perfect. And it's not enough to offset the time it takes to get produce from the orchard to your mouth.

Think about it. That apple's got to go from tree to crate to truck, and then perhaps thousands of miles to a wholesale market. Then to the retail market's loading area, then to the produce aisle, then to your refrigerator, and then to your table.

At any step along the way, it can sit in storage for days, weeks, months. What you end up eating is a mere semblance of a fruit. It's an old soldier that's been sprayed, emptied, green-harvested, gassed, dyed, waxed, trucked, and stored. Is it any wonder kids don't want to eat their fruits and vegetables?

THE FINAL INSULT

There's more. Most of the food we eat isn't fresh. (And, as we've seen, even the fresh food we eat isn't fresh.) It's processed—meaning it's been dehydrated, reconstituted, gutted, precooked, and loaded up with chemicals for any number of reasons. Then it's packaged, canned, or bottled, with chemical preservatives added in to salvage any semblance of food value. Canned green beans? It's like eating canned nothing. And it tastes like it, in my humble opinion.

Processed food is not alive. It's not alive with nutrients. It's not alive with enzymes. It's not alive with probiotics, which are the bacterial flora that your gut needs to properly break down food. Processed foods are so devoid of vitamins, minerals, phytochemicals, and other nutrients, and usually fiber as well, that some of those things are often added artificially, sometimes by law. Check your cereal box sometime.

In fact, peruse the ingredients box on the label of any processed food, from mashed potato mix to Pop-Tarts®. It looks like a nightmare homework assignment from chemistry class. Here's a rule of thumb: If you can't pronounce any of the ingredients, don't eat the food.

ORGANIC IS GREAT, BUT . . .

As a response to the problems I've been discussing, more fruits and vegetables today are being grown organically—without pesticides and without synthetic fertilizers. Thanks to the perseverance of some dedicated visionaries who knew a bad thing when they saw it, organic produce is verging on the mainstream today, although it still constitutes a minuscule percentage of the produce market.

I'm basically a conservative-establishment type, and I'll admit that I thought that the people screaming about the need for organically grown food back in the '60s and '70s were nut cases. Thank goodness they didn't listen to me.

But the organic movement hasn't solved the problem and won't for a very long time, if ever. For one thing, few people eat organic produce and that's not going to change soon. More importantly, organic farming is still subject to the same harsh realities as nonorganic farming.

Organic produce can't hide from the toxins that permeate the earth; acid rain doesn't refuse to fall on organic fields. Also, organic crops are just as affected by depleted soil as any other crop. And organic produce is often green harvested, since commercial pressures also apply to organic farmers. The distances it travels can be long. And it can be sprayed in the stores.

Most organic produce is picked even greener than "regular" produce because it doesn't have the chemicals to sustain shelf life as long as commercially grown produce. That reality is reflected in the studies I've seen, which estimate that only about 50 percent (and maybe less) of organic produce arrives at the grocery store chemical-free. I must say, though, that a 50 percent chance of getting fewer chemicals with my food is worth the higher price I usually have to pay for organic produce.

So yes, organically grown fruits and vegetables are not *as* toxic, but they can be just *as* nutritionally depleted as commercially grown produce. They are clearly preferable, especially if you can buy them at local farmers' markets or grow them yourself. But they're still toxic. And they're still depleted. Organic is not the answer.

FAT, SICK, AND DEPLETED: THE CONNECTION

To sum up: Depleted soil and premature harvesting rob our food of nutrients. So even as you eat lots of "fresh" fruits and vegetables—as you've been told you should—you're not getting the natural vitamins, minerals, enzymes, amino acids, probiotics, and phytochemicals that you should be. If you eat mostly processed foods, you're getting even less nutrition and many more toxic chemicals.

In short, you're undernourished.

I've got a hunch I know what you're thinking right about now: "Dr. Marilyn, you've convinced me that nutrient depletion is a serious problem these days. But what's that got to do with my weight?"

The answer is, "Everything."

It's no coincidence that the nutritional value of our food supply has been decreasing over the last four or five decades just as obesity has climbed its way to epidemic proportions. The truth is that poor nutrition is responsible for the excess body fat that so many Americans are carrying around.

Let me explain briefly why that is.

THE STUBBORNNESS OF CELLS

As you probably know, cells are the basic units of life. But a fact that's more important for your health and fat loss goals is that cells carry out all functions of living things. Everything that happens in your body—from your heart beating to your kidneys cleansing—takes place at the cellular level. You're able to read my words right now because cells are doing their job.

Cells are highly motivated to do what they're supposed to do. Since they can't perform without nutrients from outside the body in the form of food delivered through the bloodstream, they insist on getting nourished. If the food you eat doesn't provide enough nutrients—and you know by now that it doesn't—your cells aren't going to accept that kind of insult. They're like hungry kids; they're not going to pipe down until they get what they want.

You may be perfectly happy with that apple you picked up at the supermarket, but you can't fool cells with dyes and wax. The nutrients are either there or they're not. If they're not, your cells know it. They'll want you to eat another apple, or something else that's sweet. This craving for sweets is your body's way of telling us that you are missing the nutrients that would have made the apple sweet. That's where your problems start.

When your body's not provided with the nutrition it needs to run your system properly, it's going to keep you hungry and craving all kinds of foods. You're not conscious of it, of course, but you're getting signals that something's missing. Sooner or later, you respond to those signals by eating more.

Sometimes it's sooner, rather than later. Have you ever gotten up after a huge meal and found yourself rummaging through the cupboards or refrigerator? You're stuffed, but you're looking for more food! How can you be full and hungry at the same time? What's going on here? You're not looking for "comfort," you're looking for nutrition! What's going on is that your body is trying to keep you alive. It hasn't been nutritionally satisfied, and it's trying to rectify the matter in the only way it knows how—by demanding more food. You, in return, respond to those demands in the only way you know how—by eating more "food."

So the calories accumulate and the pounds pile on, but the nutrients are still nowhere to be found. You're overfed and undernourished.

THE SOURCE OF THE PROBLEM

Eating more apples is one response to your body's protest against that empty apple you fed it. More likely, though, you're going to eat apple pie.

Remember, you have a built-in taste for natural sweetness because it indicates a mature and nutrient-rich fruit or vegetable. Of course, pouring refined sugar over apple slices and baking them in lard-loaded pie crust isn't the kind of sweetness your body had in mind. Even though you're unconsciously trying to please your cells, you're doing it all wrong. But who can blame you? The right way—naturally nutritious food—is unavailable.

Your cells' cries for help are the true source of those diabolical cravings that have made it so hard for you to go from fat to lean by following the usual prevailing eating programs out there. I don't think much of the popular notion of "comfort foods" or the prevailing view that your cravings are an emotional response to stress. Don't for a minute let them convince you that some alleged emotional weakness is somehow responsible for your cravings. *You're* not the culprit.

The root of the problem is physical. It's the undernourishment of your cells. Emotional stress does indeed contribute to the problem—but for reasons that end up being physical as well. Stress further depletes certain nutrients in your body, and *that's* what drives you to eat certain foods even more.

I believe cravings for chocolate, peanut butter, and alcohol are all the same mechanism—just a different imbalance—that when addressed through the correct nutritional supplements can balance your system and eliminate those cravings. Any kind of craving is your body's natural response that springs out of a nutritional need. Thousands of times I've had elated, shocked clients come back in a few weeks and tell me about their cravings that have disappeared, with the additional comment of thinking that would *never* happen.

THE DOWNWARD SPIRAL

Very few people have walked into my Nashville practice with only body fat for a problem. Usually their weight issues go hand-in-hand with health problems. Some of these people are very ill, like I was. All of them are at least feeling low, draggy, never quite 100 percent.

That's certainly no surprise. The same cell undernourishment that leads to weight gain also leads to system imbalance and disease. What makes you fat makes you sick.

Just think of the task that the depleted food supply imposes on our bodies. Cells expend enormous amounts of energy breaking down food that doesn't deliver the enzymes and other nutrients needed to run that process. In the absence of those nutrients, they ask for more food. But their nutrient-starved condition makes it harder for them to process the additional food they've ordered.

Soon you're trapped in an out-of-control downward spiral that's making you sicker and fatter. Your unbalanced system, as a result of your undernourished cells, also has a hard time eliminating waste and toxins. It's not a question of junk in, junk out. It's junk in ... and staying in. Organ function—bowel, kidneys, liver, and the rest—is compromised as a result.

So there's another vicious cycle. The food we eat from plants and animals insults our systems with pesticides, herbicides, antibiotics, and growth hormones, but doesn't deliver the nutritional potency to get rid of those toxins.

In addition, constant exposure to environmental carcinogens means cancer cells are developed on a daily basis. A healthy, nutritionally balanced immune system has the power to detect and destroy these microscopic malignancies before they grow into life-threatening tumors. But the toxic nutrient-depleted food supply makes that hard to do.

YOUR MISSION: STOP STARVING YOURSELF

Let me put it bluntly: If you're twenty or more pounds overweight, you're terribly malnourished. You're slowly starving yourself to death. So what do you do about it? Well, here are three things you *can't* do about it.

◻ *You can't eat more* to stop starving yourself, since you're already overeating. Besides, the more you eat, the more imbalanced and malnourished you'll be.

□ *You can't eat better* to stop starving yourself, because the nutrient levels won't be adequate no matter what you eat. Of course you do want to eat healthier overall and consume only the calories you need (and eventually you'll be doing just that). But as a solution to the immediate problem (malnourishment), such worthy goals are irrelevant.

□ *You can't eat less* to stop starving yourself. At least, not right away. Trying now to cut your food intake in any significant way will only court frustration. The cravings that have put you in the situation you're in aren't going to disappear just because you promise yourself to eat less. That's why diets never work for long. They don't deal with the true source of your poor food choices, your tendency to overeat, and your out-of-control cravings.

That source, as we've seen, is our nutrient-depleted food supply. Your mind may be craving a certain food, but your body is craving specific nutrients that are supposed to be in that food—but aren't.

Bottom line: Your body needs nutrients, but can't get them whether you eat more, less, the same, or differently.

That certainly sounds like a problem, doesn't it?

It is THE problem. And it needs to be solved before you even think about dieting or detoxifying your system. But here's the best piece of news I've given you so far: It can be solved.

How? Well, the first order of business has to be to find some other way to nourish your starving cells. And guess what? That's exactly the first order of business in the Nashville Diet.

As you go through my program, you'll find your cravings for certain foods will diminish while your taste for healthier food increases. You'll eat less because you'll have no desire to eat more. And you'll go from fat to lean because you'll nourish your body, not deprive it.

All that won't happen because you've used willpower. It won't happen because you've follow a low-protein diet or a low-carb diet or a fat-free diet or any other kind of diet that does little more than rearrange the deck chairs on the Titanic. It will happen because the nutritional needs that were driving your cravings for too much of the wrong foods will have been met.

THE SOLUTION:

food in a capsule

the nashville diet is based on one key strategy above all others —
the daily nourishment of your body with concentrated, nutrient-rich food
taken in capsule form. I call it nutraplenishment™.

Given our nutrient-depleted, chemical-loaded food supply, nutraplenishing is the only way to provide your cells with the natural substances
they need. Therefore, it is the only way to control your food cravings, restore your metabolic efficiency, shed your excess body fat, and regain the
vibrant health that is your birthright.

The idea is worth repeating: Nutraplenishment is the *only* way to provide your cells with the nutrients they need so you can lose weight.
Without it, any diet you try is doomed to failure. Why? Because you're still
starving.

That holds true for the Nashville Diet itself. The healthy eating plan
you'll be following will take you from fat to lean, sure. But in and of itself,
it's merely a good plan on paper. You can't drive a car without gasoline,
and you can't follow a healthy, fat-to-lean eating plan without thoroughly
nourished cells. Nutraplenishing has to come first.

That's why we're not even going to get into your actual eating program until Part Three of this book. Not that healthy eating isn't important—it most definitely is. But it must be preceded by weeks, maybe even months, of nutraplenishing. And you need to continue your nutraplenishing even as you adjust your eating patterns.

In fact, nutraplenishing via concentrated, capsulated food is a permanent necessity in today's world, even after you achieve your ideal weight. Your systems' need for natural vitamins, minerals, enzymes, probiotics, amino acids, and myriad phytochemicals doesn't disappear along with the unwanted body fat. You have to continue to fill your car up with gas in order to drive it. Nor are those nutrients ever going to reappear in the food we eat, at least not in our lifetime. You need to keep getting them in concentrated form. Nutraplenishing is a lifelong health and weight control strategy.

In the June 19, 2002, issue of *The Journal of the American Medical Association* (JAMA) your doctor's monthly "bible," the old thought of "eat right and exercise" was put to rest as the article cited years of studies showing that taking nutritional supplements should now be recommended by your doctor.

With so many supplements on the market, and a new fad supplement or diet coming out every week, the Nashville Diet will lead you through this jungle to a good-quality plan of supplements that will truly make a difference in your health and weight—permanently.

ADDITION BY EXTRACTION

Not long ago I was taken out to one of those trendy Mongolian-style food bars—the kind of place where people tend to overindulge. The food was indeed good, and I enjoyed a nice meal.

But you know what? I didn't really eat all that much, though there was plenty available. Good as it was, the food wasn't all that important to me. I had some, appreciated it, and moved on to other things besides dining. This is now a way of life for me and all of my clients who have been "converted" to real vibrant health. If we'd been told upon entering the restaurant that the kitchen had just closed and we couldn't be served, I wouldn't have been upset at all. It just didn't matter to me that much.

There was a time in my life when I would have marched into that restaurant with an outsized hunger, eager to try every exotic dish on the menu. Sound familiar? For me, the difference between then and now is that now I'm nutritionally satisfied because I've been taking my nutrients in capsule form every day for years. I don't need to eat so much. And because my body is no longer constantly demanding missing nutrition, I don't eat more than I need.

The best part is that now I find it so easy to eat only healthy food. If I have no particular urge to indulge in rich, heavy food, such as the Mongolian delicacies at that restaurant, you can imagine how little the unhealthy stuff appeals to me. I simply don't want bad food; after all these years, I can literally taste the chemicals. I won't eat any food that I know is going to make me feel bad. I'd just as soon not eat. Someone told me I was going to be like that along the way. I never believed it, but it's true for me and will be for you too, if you follow the Nashville Diet.

That's what nutraplenishing will do for you. You won't have to "resist" eating unhealthy food or any food in unhealthy amounts. You just won't want it. When your cells' nutrient requirements are fulfilled, your physical appetite will finally cooperate with your mental knowledge of what's good (and bad) for you.

For example, I don't need to tell you that eating greasy junk food is unhealthy. You already know that. Still, if you've been hitting the fast-food joints all you're life, you're not going to stop just because I tell you to. You already know that. But you *will* stop if you no longer have any desire for the stuff. And that's exactly what happens when you nourish your cells with concentrated nutrients.

As you become more nourished (and detoxified, as you'll learn in Part Two), your cravings will change completely. As of now, you've become desensitized to the chemicals and hormones in the foods you eat. But once you nutraplenish and detoxify, not only will you not want the foods you're now addicted to, you won't even be able to stand eating them.

Personally, I can't stand the smell of fast-food places. I'd rather eat a piece of fruit and drink some clean water than eat in some of those places. Not because I know the fruit and water are better for my health, but because I truly *prefer* them.

I have a new client named Samuel who came in very worried about his fast-food fried chicken addiction. Samuel's biggest concern was that he'd never be able to "give this up." I told him not to try to quit his fried chicken habit cold turkey, so to speak. Instead, I encouraged him to not even try to stop eating the stuff for the first three weeks. A better strategy was to give his body some real nutrition via nutraplenishing and let the supplements do that part of the hard work for him.

Sure enough, Samuel called me the first time he visited his favorite fried chicken fast-food restaurant after he'd started nutraplenishing. He told me, "I can't believe it! Not only did I only eat one and a half pieces instead of my usual full bucket, but I didn't want it!" He was on his way to vibrant health. Samuel went on to talk about how energetic he now feels, and the mental clarity was unbelievable to him. Samuel has shrunk four pants sizes so far and has put his sixty-five-year-old father on the Nashville Diet. Now they both call me, laughing about how they're both running circles around men half their age on their job site. Samuel also talks about what a good mood he's in. (Here's your chance, ladies, to get that man in your life in a better mood! Get him started on losing weight and you'll have a leaner, happier man in your life!).

With nutraplenishing, there's no longer any reason to overeat or to eat what you shouldn't.

So you don't. Just like Samuel didn't.

It's that simple.

GETTING LEAN AND HEALTHY TOGETHER

Talking about fat loss without talking about improved health is meaningless. It's also dangerous. After all, you can drop plenty of pounds by losing yourself in the Arizona desert for a few weeks. But there's no best-selling book called The Get-Lost-in-the-Desert 40-Day-and-40-Night Diet Miracle because few would consider it worth the risk.

Sadly, though, similar risks are taken every day by well-meaning people on impossible calorie-deprivation diets who are literally trying to starve themselves thin. They are doing nothing to nourish their cells, so they're doing nothing to correct the health issue that underlies their body-fat problems. That underlying issue is poor cell function that results from undernourishment. Eventually, of course, the angry cries of the famished cells are going to overwhelm the willpower that these poor dieters depend on to eat less. Then the binge parade starts. The infamous yo-yo diet syndrome is in full gear.

Nutraplenishing comes at your problem in a completely different way. Instead of trying to *subtract* something (calories) from your life, it *adds* what's missing (nutrients). That addition cuts your food cravings. But as it cuts those cravings and decreases your appetite, in general, it also restores your cells' abilities to perform tasks that are essential for good health. In fact, the very *reason* you lose your cravings is because your cells are now better able to perform those tasks. Quite literally, you're getting leaner because you're getting healthier.

When you nourish your cells with highly concentrated natural nutrients, you're giving them what they need to:

- Build up your immune system to fight off disease.
- Replenish your intestinal flora and enzymatic systems for better digestion.
- Purge your system of excess waste.
- Eliminate harmful toxins, such as parasites, candida, chemicals, and carcinogens.
- Keep your hormonal system in balance.
- Boost your metabolism.

Looked at from the opposite direction, the absence of adequate nutrition limits your cells' ability to get those vital jobs done. As a result, your

body is not in a healthy balance. Is it any wonder the cells insist on getting the nutrients they need, making their wishes known by triggering a
process that results in hunger and cravings?

You have three choices for dealing with the demands of those undernourished, poorly functioning cells:

1. You can give in to the hunger and cravings by eating more.
   The excess nutrient-deleted food won't meet your cells'
   needs, and it won't improve your health, but it will keep
   you fat, overloaded, and out of balance.

2. You can try to conquer the hunger and cravings by following any one of a million calorie-restriction diets. You
   still won't be meeting your cells' needs, you'll do little for
   your health, and you'll soon gain back any weight you're
   able to lose.

3. You can nourish your cells with daily capsules of concentrated, nutrient-rich food. You'll meet your cells' needs,
   improve your health, and eliminate the hunger and cravings so you can shed body fat and return to your natural
   weight by eating reasonable amounts of healthy food.

I find that an easy choice to make. Don't you?

NUTRIENTS FOR HEALTH: THE CASE OF CALCIUM

There's not really any doubt left that nutrition is critical in maintaining
wellness and preventing disease. Half of all diseases in the United States
are related to nutritional factors. Most can be either prevented or treated
with proper nutrition.

I've explained how poor nutrition affects your body systemically—in
other words, how undernourished cells compromise such key functions
as metabolism and waste elimination. I've also pointed out how inadequate nutrition limits your immune system's ability to attack the cancer

cells that are constantly being formed in your body. Now let me illustrate how vital it is to take your nutrients in concentrated form by giving you a thumbnail example of how an inadequate supply and the wrong form of just one nutrient can lead to a specific disease.

You're probably familiar with calcium. It's a mineral that's used in all cells. But your body is such a miraculous creation that it will prioritize its use of calcium (or any other nutrient) to sustain life. That means, in this case, that your heart gets first dibs on any available calcium.

Why? Because calcium plays a role in regulating the electrical flow that controls your heartbeat. Each heart cell beats independently, but at the same time they all work together to maintain a perfect, life-giving pulse—the beating of your heart. To make that happen, a perfect balance of calcium must be present at all times in every heart cell.

If that balance is off just a smidgeon, the electrical impulses get thrown out of kilter and sections of your heart may beat out of rhythm. This fibrillation, as it's called, can lead to cardiac arrest and death.

Fortunately, your body isn't inclined to let such a thing happen. To make sure that your cardiac cells always have enough calcium, it gives top priority to maintaining a proper calcium balance in the bloodstream, the feeder of all cells. That balance—of calcium and every other vital substance—is called homeostasis.

But say you're not getting enough calcium in your diet to maintain that balance (which is probably the case). What then? Well, your body's going to get that calcium into the bloodstream one way or another. We're talking about a matter of life and death here. And just as John Dillinger said he robbed banks because that's where the money is, your bloodstream robs your bones because that's where the calcium is.

And you know what that means—osteoporosis, the weakening of your bones. As disturbing as the thought may be, osteoporosis is actually a life-saving mechanism. Your bones have sacrificed calcium for the greater good, namely the continued beating of your heart. Blood tests will show that your calcium supply is fine, because the blood level is indeed adequate. But overall, you're calcium-deficient.

FOOD IN A CAPSULE

Have you noticed that I've avoided using the familiar term *supplements* to describe the concentrated nutrients in capsule form that are at the heart of the Nashville Diet? In truth, supplementation is exactly what you'll be doing every day. You'll be *supplementing* your nutrient-depleted food with nutrients in a concentrated form, taken in capsules.

But the word supplement usually conjures up a pill-taking routine that has little to do with the kind of nutraplenishing you need to feed your cells and get on the road to recovery. New clients of mine often tell me, "But Dr. Tucker, I'm already supplementing every day!" Which usually means they're swallowing a multiple vitamin, perhaps with calcium and iron, and maybe even an herb or two they've read about, like ginkgo or ginseng.

That's like shooting in the dark with the wrong kind of bullets. Your cells need to be replenished with the right amounts of *all* of the most important nutrients that they're not getting from food. And they need those nutrients in the right form.

Run-of-the-mill commercial supplements rarely meet those criteria.

So, yes, you do need to supplement. But with what? The answer to that question is the foundation of the Nashville Diet. It doesn't require a degree in pharmacology, but it does require mastering a new learning curve. That's what I'm going to help you do.

NUTRACEUTICALS TO THE RESCUE

The supplements you'll be taking to help you move from fat to lean fall under a whole new realm of healing agents called nutraceuticals. A nutraceutical is a nutrient with a pharmaceutical action. It is nutrition as medicine. While a pharmaceutical drug may sometimes be inspired by a naturally occurring substance, it is almost always synthetic. A nutraceutical, on the other hand, is always 100 percent natural or, to put it a better way, from living plants—it's alive. You must have living food to keep you alive.

Nutraceuticals can be vitamins, minerals, or herbs. They can be enzymes, like CoQ-10. They can be plant hormones (phytoestrogens), like genistein from soybeans. They can be amino acids, like glutamine or tyrosine. They can belong to numerous classes of plant compounds (phytochemicals), such as bioflavonoids (like quercetin), carotenoids (like beta-carotene), and polyphenols (like curcumin).

They can be lots of things. But they cannot be synthetic. Synthetic implies something made in a chemistry lab, something not living. If it's not natural, it's not a neutraceutical.

That sets your nutraceuticals apart from the synthetic vitamins and minerals that rule the supplement market. Synthetic vitamins are chemicals manufactured in a laboratory, just like any other pharmaceutical drug. They're designed to mimic the real thing, but they're not the real thing.

For example, typical vitamin C tablets are made from ascorbic acid. But ascorbic acid is not the vitamin C you find in limes or oranges—or at least in those limes and oranges that aren't grown in weak soil, oversprayed, chemically fertilized, and green harvested.

So even though supermarket aisles are bursting with a dizzying selection of supplements, most of them aren't doing a whole lot for anybody. At the cellular level, our bodies are no more fooled by synthetic supplements than they are by depleted produce.

Nutraceuticals, on the other hand, are concentrated nutrients extracted mainly from plants that are specially grown and selected for their rich nutritional value. When you get right down to it, nutraceuticals are food. Each time you supplement with them, you're having a meal. It's a meal without much in the way of calories, to be sure, but with more beneficial nutrients in it than you'd get from eating an entire salad bar.

That's what nutraceuticals are—real nutrients extracted from the active components of real living food, concentrated down and put into capsules. Because of that process, your cells recognize what they're getting as bona fide nutrients. They accept them, they use them, and after a certain amount of time they stop behaving like deprived stepchildren. They call off the cravings, and you're ready to shed fat and feel great.

Eating Rocks Is a Bad Idea, Isn't It?

To give you an idea of the importance of getting your nutrients in the right form, let's go back to our old friend calcium. The best primary sources for this vital mineral (rather than having it go through animals and then be consumed as dairy products) are carrots and dark-green leafy vegetables like spinach, mustard greens, and broccoli. However, our theme holds true here. When you buy those vegetables—fresh or frozen—they're very unlikely to provide for you the calcium they did once upon a time. These days you'd have to juice a ton of the stuff to get enough calcium in you. Would you want to do that every day? I sure wouldn't.

So it's important for you to supplement with calcium, which is what about 25 percent of American women do. But how are they getting that calcium? For the most part, calcium's delivered in the form of calcium carbonate, which is essentially ground-up limestone. I'm not exaggerating—the same limestone used in brick manufacturing is used in most of the calcium supplements on the market today. The most popular antacid is actually what we would call chewable calcium carbonate. The antacid manufacturers get their raw materials to produce all those tablets from one of the largest brick manufacturers in the United States. And yes, it is the same material they use in the brick process. The raw materials only cost about $50 per ton, about a boxcar-full on a freight train. So when you buy these "rocks"—calcium carbonate supplements—you're literally paying over 95 percent for packaging and marketing for the privilege of taking flavored or encapsulated rocks.

Not surprisingly, your cells aren't inclined to absorb calcium in this form. On the molecular level, calcium carbonate is very different from the calcium complexes found naturally in green vegetables. The plant molecules form a matrix that's like a twisted strand of pearls. The cells recognize that matrix as food, so it becomes the key that opens the cell "door." The calcium carbonate key doesn't fit in that lock.

Your body can't process rocks. So it's no surprise that it can't process calcium carbonate. It needs calcium from plants. The only way to get that form of calcium is from nutraceuticals that consist of highly concentrated extracts from such calcium-containing vegetables as broccoli, Brussels sprouts, carrots, and cauliflower. That's one kind of nutraceutical I'll be recommending to you as you embark on the Nashville Diet. And, of course, such a concentrated vegetable supplement will provide you with much more in the way of plant-based nutrients than just calcium.

NOT JUST ANY OLD SUPPLEMENT WILL DO

In the best of all possible worlds, we'd get the nutrients we need from organically grown fruits, vegetables, grains, fish, and (for most people) meat. We'd eat like Adam and Eve did, and we'd all be nourished, healthy, lean, and gorgeous. But we no longer live in such a world. Our food supply is nutrient-depleted, so we have to nutraplenish instead.

In the second-best of all possible worlds, we'd at least have a host of natural and effective supplements easily available to us for our nutraplenishing. But most of what's out there is synthetic and/or incompatible with our cellular requirements. So we need to search out nutraceuticals.

In the third-best of all possible worlds, the nutraceuticals would be of uniformly good quality and deliver the health benefits they're supposed to. But nutraceuticals are still a new phenomenon, so they vary in quality, potency, and effectiveness. For our nutraplenishing to get the job done, we have to use not just the *right* nutraceuticals, but the highest *quality* nutraceuticals.

Why is quality so important? Because nutraceuticals are by definition created from real food components. If the original food from which they're extracted suffers from any of the nutrient-depleting practices we've been learning about—depleted soil, green harvesting, spraying, long shelf-life, and so on—then those neutraceuticals will be practically worthless to you.

What's more, the way the nutraceuticals are manufactured can either preserve or compromise their effectiveness. There's a lot involved in getting those nutrients out of the plant and into your capsules. If these products are not properly grown, harvested, dried, tested, and processed, you end up with minimal nutritional value.

Finally, the federal government doesn't regulate nutritional supplements as it does pharmaceuticals, so quality standards have to come voluntarily from the manufacturers themselves. Needless to say, some are more conscientious about it than others.

Later on, in Chapter Four, I will be giving you some pointers on how to pick a quality product from a good, reliable manufacturer.

SECRETS OF A POWERFUL NUTRACEUTICAL

As you start to nutraplenish for health and weight loss, you're putting yourself on the cutting edge of nutrition. As a pioneer, you don't have the advantage of a well-worn trail, with abundant information at your fingertips. That's why the "learning curve" I mentioned earlier is so important. Know your nutrients!

But you're not on your own. As a pharmacist who has personally taken everything I recommend and who has experience with thousands of clients, I have developed some nutraplenishing strategies that can restore you to optimal health and weight. I've dedicated myself to promoting the use of quality nutraceuticals. After all, they saved my life. You and I are in this together.

So let's take a look at some of the "musts" that differentiate a nutraceutical you'll be taking from a run-of-the-mill commercial supplement.

It must come from properly harvested plants. As I've already pointed out, nutraceutical components can only be effective if they're extracted from plants grown in nutrient-rich soil, spared contamination from pesticides, and harvested at the proper time in the proper way. Otherwise, you'll have the same problems you have with nutrient-depleted "regular" food.

It must come from the right species. Different species of the same plant genus can have different properties. For example, Siberian ginseng and panax (or American) ginseng are two completely distinct species (not even from the same genus, in fact), and each has different effects. (As it turns out, I'll be recommending both ginsengs to you in the next chapter, but the point remains.) One raw-materials supplier I'm familiar with has over forty different kinds of green tea. Some are high in antioxidant properties with little to no caffeine, while others are high in caffeine with little to no antioxidant effect. Sometimes manufacturers aren't as diligent as they should be in making sure they've been shipped the right species to work with. Many consumers don't care, but we nutra-plenishers care a lot. That's why we're careful label readers and fussy about the products we buy.

It must come from the right part of the plant. This is a key factor in the formulation of a nutraceutical that will work. The active component may be best concentrated in the roots, the leaves, the bark, the fruit, the flowers, or a number of other plant parts. It depends on the nutrients you want and the plant you're getting it from. For example, the dried and concentrated broccoli I'll be recommending should come from the flowering head. The wild yam, however, must be a root extract. The elderberry extract you need comes from the fruit itself. In many cases, a specific nutrient is best extracted from mere sprouts of the plant, since sprouts often offer a tremendously concentrated source of nutrients.

It must be dried with care. Plant extracts need to be dehydrated to get them into capsules in concentrated form. But the willy-nilly techniques that all too often plague the supplement industry can rob the product of its properties. Some plant extracts need to be dried in the dark, because the ultraviolet rays of the sun will deactivate the key components. Others need the ultraviolet light to activate the components. Some plant ingredients will perish with too-high temperatures. A manufacturer of quality pharmaceuticals won't accept raw materials that haven't been dehydrated in a way that preserves their potency.

It must be tested for quality. There's no law requiring nutraceutical manufacturers to test their products for efficacy. The supplier of the raw material will usually provide a certificate of authenticity, promising that the substance is indeed what was ordered and free of E. coli or other bacteria. Most manufacturers that I've inspected simply take that piece of paper (which is all it is) at face value, and then slap the stuff in capsules and send it out the door. But the best companies will voluntarily test throughout the process. They need to get samples in the lab to make sure that they got what they asked for (the right species from the right part of the plant), and to make sure that the potency and concentration are what they should be.

You Deserve the Best

All of what I just ran down for you sounds a bit complicated, I know. But I certainly don't mean to paint you a gloomy picture of unattainable standards for the nutraceuticals you need for nutraplenishing. On the contrary, I want you to understand the difference between nutraplenishing with potent, high-quality nutraceuticals and mere "supplementation." That difference is so very important for achieving your weight-loss goals.

What you need is out there. And I'm here to see that you get it, as I share with you my knowledge of nutraceuticals and guide you through your nutraplenishing program. And believe me, there's nothing I love more in the world than making people like you aware of what they can do to turn their lives around—finally!

The nutrition you put into your body represents one of the most far-reaching decisoins you will ever make. The formulas, quality, purity, and potency of your nutraceuticals and food are critical for your success. The Vibrant Health Seal of Approval© was created because of widespread lack of quality controls within the food and nutraceutical industries.

The Vibrant Health Seal of Approval assures you that the recommended products and foods have been examined and passed my minimum requirements for quality, purity, and potency. Since this is such a dynamic industry, with changes happening daily, look for the most current list of approved products at www.NashvilleDiet.com or call 1-866-Dr-Tucker (1-866-378-8253).

In the next chapter, I'm going to go over, one by one, all the nutraceuticals you should be taking, and what to look for to make sure you're getting the good stuff. Then I'm going to outline for you an easy-to-follow program for taking them.

Before you know it, you'll be nutraplenishing your way to a new, leaner you!

the nutrients you need

as you embark on your journey to vibrant health, I want
you to be aware of one solemn truth that I just can't emphasize enough.
You cannot lose weight by taking a pill. Just banish the idea from your
mind. That's the old fad-diet mentality. The nutrient supplements that
form the foundation of the Nashville Diet are not weight-loss pills. They're
concentrated food that delivers long-lost nutrients to your cells.

The Nashville Diet puts you at your desired weight because this re-
nourishing of your cells improves the functioning of your internal systems
and eliminates cravings so you can resume healthy eating habits as your
body more efficiently processes your food.

You'll also be helping this health-reviving process along by taking
action to detoxify your body and by learning to make the right kind of
food choices. But before those important steps are taken, you first must
nutraplenish.

Which leads to a logical question: What do you nutraplenish *with*?

Well, as you're about to see, with lots of things. Over years of helping
desperate clients so nutrient-poor that they'd just about given up on ever

regaining their figure or their health, I've put together an optimal nutra-plenishing program. It wasn't easy. It took a lot of trial and error and ar-duous research to pull together a line-up of nutrients with a broad enough array of actions. But what I came up with works. Consistent nutraplen-ishing with the quality-tested nutraceuticals I describe in this chapter will bring balance to your systems.

But here's another important concept about nutraplenishing. The nu-trients themselves do not balance any system. Instead, they give your body the missing raw materials it needs to balance itself. And they're not drugs. They don't eliminate symptoms of poor health. Rather, they bring nour-ishment so your body is able to heal itself.

In other words, nutraplenishing gives you the means to take charge of your own health and fat loss.

That does not mean, of course, that your nutraceuticals replace any need for conventional medicine that you might have now. Some health issues need to be addressed by medications and other remedies, such as surgery, under a physician's guidance. But that's an even stronger reason to strengthen your system with these incredible nutrients. Just keep your doctor informed about what you're taking. Please do not attempt to adjust or change your prescription medications without your doctor's knowledge and advice.

NUTRIENTS FOR EVERY OCCASION

The first thing you'll probably notice about the list of nutrients I'm rec-ommending is how long it is. Don't let this intimidate you. These are the supplements you need to do the job your nutrient-depleted food isn't doing, and to reap lots of important health benefits as well. You'll soon learn to love every one of these nutrients. But there's no denying a cen-tral fact about the Nashville Diet: You'll be taking some capsules every day. And you'll have to plan on spending some money to get them. Trust me, you're worth it.

One reason there are so many players in your nutrient line-up is the variety of benefits you'll be getting. You need a *complete* system of nourishment. So I've included a number of different kinds of nutrients that work in a number of different ways and help a number of different systems in your body.

Some of the nutrients work to strengthen your immune system. Some boost your metabolism, which is so vital to fat loss. Some help balance your hormonal system. Some target your gastrointestinal tract to improve your digestion and eliminate toxins.

I've categorized your nutrients according to their principal actions. But keep in mind that most pack multiple benefits that cross the boundaries of the categories.

THE RIGHT STUFF

I've explained how the quality of a nutrient supplement can vary widely from product to product. There's no hiding the fact that it's hard to find the well-processed stuff, or to know it when you see it. Now that you'll actually be looking to buy some nutraceuticals, this challenge is an immediate concern to you.

In the nutrient descriptions that follow, I'm including where possible any information that will help you know what to look for and which bottle from the store shelf to take home. But much of your success is up to you. You'll need to start honing your knowledge of supplements so you can make good decisions about the products you buy.

I know that sounds out of the question to you right now. Just the whole idea of nutraplenishing might seem bewildering at first, especially as you read through all the nutrients listed below. But you'd be surprised at how much knowledge about a subject you can accumulate when you're personally involved with it. And I guarantee you, once you start feeling what these nutrients do for your health, you're going to be interested in learning more. It will be a pleasure.

Besides, this "hands-on" approach validates your commitment to your health. Remember, you're not just popping pills to lose weight. You're nourishing your cells with concentrated food. I urge you to become involved in the "whys" and "hows" of your weight loss strategies, and not just blindly follow instructions. Learning about the details of these wonderful natural nutrients is an important part of your involvement. You became knowledgeable about which food products to buy, didn't you? Now you can also become knowledgeable about what nutritional supplements are best. Just walk into a good health-food store and start looking around. Here are some tips to get you started.

Become a label reader. The name of the product often doesn't clearly indicate what's actually in the capsules. The small-print ingredients section on the label will tell you much more about what you need to know. Watch out for products that use the name of a nutrient but actually offer very little of it and a lot of extraneous ingredients.

Browse before you buy. Compare the labels of lots of different brands offering the same product. Not only will that help you find the best product, you'll also learn a lot.

Pay special attention to blends. Blends of different nutrients are at least as common on the shelves as single-ingredient products. You'll usually be looking for capsules containing just one plant extract or nutrient, but if more than one of the nutrients you'll be taking appear in a single product, by all means take advantage of that convenience. Just make sure you're getting enough of the nutrients you do want, and not wasting money on a whole slew of ingredients you don't need.

Keep up-to-date. The nutraceutical world is an ever-changing one. Being knowledgeable will make it easier to find the best products and make sense of the ingredients lists on the bottles. (Food and chemical companies have become more and more adept at hiding what is actually in their products.) Find good sources of news updates about health and weight-loss issues. Responsible Internet sites are plentiful, and can be updated at a moment's notice. But beware the sites that make exaggerated claims about products they're selling.

Get to know an expert. This is probably the most important advice of all. If you have access to a true expert, bring him or her with you to the health food store. Or try to find a health food store that has a knowledgeable person running the supplement section with whom you can discuss your needs and your concerns about quality. It really helps to have somebody like that on your side. And don't be shy. Tell your expert about your nutraplenishing plan and solicit his or her help in finding products for it that meet my requirements.

Of course, the ideal expert to answer your questions about nutraceuticals would be a pharmacist from your community pharmacy. Such a qualified professional would have a much better background for helping you out, assuming they have an interest in nutraceuticals. (And more and more pharmacists are interested; in fact, the last three continuing education seminars I've attended featured discussions of nutritional supplements and vitamins.)

Still, most of us in the pharmacy field have been educated to give a chemical solution to any problem. Since chemicals are exactly what you want to avoid, have a short, exploratory conversation with your pharmacist to test his or her attitude about nutraceuticals. A good test question might be about the difference between ascorbic acid and vitamin C, or between calcium carbonate and calcium in food. If your pharmacist doesn't consider the difference significant, he or she probably won't be much help in your nutraceutical quest.

Now let's look at our nutraceuticals.

The Immune Boosters

All your nutrients are vital, but the three key ingredients in your nutraplenishing regimen are first among equals. You might already be familiar with one of them — aloe vera. The other two have rather intimidating-sounding names that you'll learn to love sooner than you think. All three of them are wonderful natural substances that I've seen bring incredible benefits to client after client of mine. I absolutely love these three nutrients. They literally saved my life. They're manna for your immune system, which is your body's defense against infectious disease, toxins, cancer cell formation, and other unwelcome invaders. Remember, if you're overweight, you can be sure that your immune system is seriously compromised by undernourishment, toxic overload, pharmaceutical drugs, and other assorted ills of modern life. It needs the help that these immune boosters deliver. And it needs it every day.

Aloe vera. This miraculous succulent plant is well known for healing burns and as an anti-aging agent in skin creams. But its nutra-plenishing value goes way beyond those topical uses. The aloe vera you'll be consuming every day will be in a highly concentrated form that delivers all of the numerous active biological compounds exactly as they're found in the living plant.

Those ingredients have been compared to a finely tuned orchestra, working together to deliver the kind of benefits you're looking for. The main benefit is an overall enhancement of your immune system func-tioning, including an increased capacity to fight off viral infections. Also, some studies have indicated a link between aloe vera and a reduced risk of heart disease. It certainly provides a heart-healthy cell-cleaning antiox-idant effect, since a number of the aloe vera orchestra's "instruments"—such as vitamin C, vitamin E, zinc, and seven enzymes in the superoxide dismutase category—are potent antioxidants.

Unfortunately, aloe vera is often processed in such a way that most of the key active components are degraded, rendering the product useless. So your smart-shopping skills are especially important here. Two things to insist on: One, the powder in the capsule must contain all the original plant compounds—especially the polysaccharides—and not just a "key" ingredient like aloin. Two, it must be very highly concentrated. Keep in mind that the active solids account for just a minuscule percentage of the original aloe vera gel. The rest is water. That's why I want you to make sure to take an aloe vera that's been concentrated by a factor of two hun-dred, which will show up on the label as "200:1."

Arabinogalactan. If we think of aloe vera as an orchestra of two hundred instruments, then arabinogalactan is a soloist. Called AG for short, it's a natural polysaccharide (a kind of carbohydrate) that's structurally similar to the polysaccharides that are so important in aloe vera. AG is found in lots of different plants, most notably in the bark of the larch tree, where it's thought to be responsible for the proven immune-boosting properties of that popular herb. That should give you a pretty good idea of why I'm so big on it for nutraplenishing.

AG enhances your immune system over the long haul, rather than just on an as-needed basis. And it has another major beneficial effect as a digestion aid. AG promotes the growth of "friendly" bacteria in the digestive tract, helping to get things moving through the colon (and reducing the risk of colon cancer as well). It's a fine source of dietary fiber, and as such will help you eat more sensibly by making you feel more full, since you'll take it before a meal. The encapsulated AG you'll find in health food stores will probably be extracted from the larch tree. That's what we want.

Methylsulfonylmethane (MSM). MSM is an organic compound from fruits, vegetables, grains, and (in small amounts) animals, including humans. What it delivers is sulfur, a very key element for your cellular health. Best of all, it delivers that sulfur in the friendly form of sulfonyl, which your body recognizes as food. That is definitely not the case with more harmful sulfur derivatives, such as the sulfites and sulfates used as food preservatives. Sulfa drugs are completely different and there is not usually any cross-sensitivity.

Why does your body need sulfur? For lots of reasons. One is that sulfur is a key player your body's natural detoxification process. But the most important reason is that sulfur is absolutely essential for the creation of healthy new cells. When you supplement with MSM, you're providing the sulfur needed to create enough of the two sulfur-containing amino acids (methionine and cysteine) that function as building blocks. Otherwise, a diet deficient in sulfur (which is very often the case, especially as you grow older) inhibits the growth of healthy cells, which in turn leads to disease.

MSM is a purer and simpler relative of another popular supplement, DMSO. In fact, the reason you'll be able to find MSM easily in health food stores or drugstores is because modern chemistry has found a way to separate MSM from DMSO, leaving the foul-smelling chemicals behind and crystallizing natural MSM into a form that can be stored in capsules.

FREGETABLES

"Fregetables" is my invented name for capsules of powdered vegetables and fruits that contain in concentrated form every nutrient that the plant would offer if it were full and fresh (and not depleted). In other words, you can buy vegetable capsules that have been carefully put together to deliver what real vegetables are supposed to—that is, enough amino acids, vitamins, minerals, enzymes, and specific phytonutrients that nourish your cells. They are completely natural.

The Fregetables I'm recommending here go right to the heart of what nutraplenishing is all about. Although it's sometimes a good idea to supplement with a specific mineral or other nutrient, the ideal way to get nutrients into your body is in food form. And that's just what Fregetables are—*food*. But they're food so highly concentrated that just a daily dose of the ones I'm suggesting will almost complete the "five a day" servings of fruits and vegetables recommended by the American Cancer Society.

If you've been juicing, concentrated powdered vegetables offer a convenient alternative. Juicing is a popular trend and it does deliver health benefits. But what you're juicing is still grown in depleted soil and green harvested. You need to juice a lot of produce to get significant nutrition. I juice on occasion, but after I buy and wash the fruits and vegetables, run the juicer and then clean up the mess, I usually find myself saying, "I could have had a Fregetable!"

Each of the concentrated fruit and vegetable capsules that you'll be taking provides its own specific benefits. But they *all* assist in detoxifying your systems, supporting the immune response, protecting against cancer, reducing the inflammatory responses associated with allergies, and really increasing strength and energy.

So let's take a look at the line-up of Fregetables for your nutraplenishing program. They come in three categories.

ANTIOXIDANT-RICH FREGETABLES

Free radicals are harmful oxygen molecules generated as a by-product of chemical reactions in cells. The list of woes connected to these rogue molecules is a long one, and includes asthma, allergies, weak immunity, muscle and bone damage, cataracts, cancer, and cardiovascular disease.

Why would nature allow for such harmful things to be created by necessary cell activity, such as breaking down food? Because nature also provides for getting rid of them, via nutrients that act as antioxidants. The following four Fregetables for your nutraplenishing program are loaded with antioxidant phytonutrients.

Carrot. The star antioxidant in your powdered carrot capsules is beta-carotene, a powerful member of the carotenoid group of phytochemicals that give green, red, yellow, and (in this case) orange vegetables their pigmentation.

Carotenoids act as antioxidants in the plant itself, protecting it from the free radicals released during photosynthesis. The beta-carotene and other carotenoids in carrots protect you in the same way, and act as an anticarcinogen. And beta-carotene converts to vitamin A in your body, making your carrot Fregetables a wonderful source of that important vitamin.

Beta-carotene is by no means the only beneficial carotenoid in carrots. You'll also get alpha- and gamma-carotene, lycopene, and lutein.

Tomato. The major carotenoid in tomatoes is lycopene. Like beta-carotene, it's a strong antioxidant and a cancer-fighter, especially prostate cancer. Tomatoes also deliver vitamin C (another antioxidant), the carotenoids beta-zeacarotene and lutein, and phytonutrients in another category called flavonoids. It's been shown that antioxidants like vitamin E, vitamin C, and the carotenoids work well together as a team. That's another reason why I recommend the whole fruit or vegetable as a Fregetable rather than the extracts of beta-carotene or lycopene that you see on the health food store shelves.

Blueberry or Elderberry. The antioxidant effect of these berries comes from a group of flavonoids called anthocyanidins. These are the natural chemicals responsible for the blue, purple, and red colors of fruits. Anthocyanidins support connective-tissue regeneration, increase blood flow, act as anti-inflammatory agents, and help fight off viral infections.

CRUCIFEROUS VEGETABLES

Tired of being told "Eat your broccoli"? I'm going to tell you something different. *Swallow* your broccoli. In a capsule. Along with it, swallow Brussels sprouts, cabbage, kale, and turnip root.

These are all vegetables in the "cruciferous" family, and they're chock-full of powerful health benefits. Topping the list is their ability to help your liver get rid of toxins, thanks to their high content of sulfur-containing compounds called sulforaphanes that stimulate detoxification enzymes. They're also rich in nitrogen-containing phytonutrients called indoles, which are effective anticancer weapons.

Above and beyond these specific detox benefits, cruciferous vegetables are ideal for nutraplenishing because they deliver plenty of other phytonutrients, as well as vitamins and minerals, such as vitamins A and C, and potassium and calcium. Remember, this is the way you want to get your vitamins and minerals if you can—from natural food sources.

The best cruciferous vegetable nutraceuticals are concentrated from the young sprouts, which contain twenty to fifty times more sulforaphane than the mature plants. You'll probably be able to find all or most of my recommended cruciferous Fregetables in a blend, so you don't have to buy so many different products.

PINEAPPLE AND PAPAYA

These two semi-exotic (to us) fruits have long histories as folk medicine and today we think we know why. Both offer rich doses of proteolytic enzymes, the kind that break down proteins. They aid digestion, detoxify cells, stimulate the immune system, control allergies, resist cancer, and even improve the texture of your skin. What more can you ask for?

The clients that closely adhere to the full regimen you will be learning about get what we refer to as the "vibrant health glow," as it was so aptly named by one of my clients. That's this youthful glow that can come only from the inside out. No amount of make-up or surgery will yield this same result. One morning recently I got up very early in the morning to run to the grocery store to buy some watermelon for breakfast. When the poor clerk asked, "How are you?" I said, "Great." To which she replied, "No one is great at four-thirty in the morning!" I said, "I am." She said, "I can see that. You're just one of those irritating happy little people." I went on to explain how that wasn't always the case and how she too could be "an irritating happy little person." She then remarked how I was "actually glowing" and she could see I had no make-up on. And how that was fine for me but I was thirty years younger than her. It turned out that I was in fact four years younger than her. Anyone can be young and vibrant-looking and -feeling if you just finish this course and stay with it. Hang in there and one day you too will be "an irritating happy little person." Keep going and before long you too will be glowing. The "vibrant health glow" is usually one of the first things the people around you notice and begin to comment on.

Most of us enjoy eating real pineapples and papaya. We enjoy them even though the ones we eat are puny approximations to the real, nutrient-rich versions that are still to be found in just a few places on earth. In my professional pursuit of good nutrition, I interact with folks from all over the world. And I've learned that in Africa there are pineapples so much bigger and sweeter and more nutrient-rich than those we consume in North America that you'd hardly consider them the same fruit.

So to get these fruits' nutrients in the amounts we want, we need nutraceuticals. You can find lots of products offering these enzymes extracted from the rest of the fruit. They're known as bromelain in the case of pineapple and papain in papaya. But I want you to look for capsules with a concentration of the whole fruit. That's because pineapple and papaya have more to offer than just the enzymes, including vitamin C and other antioxidant phytonutrients. It's been shown that the enzymes act synergistically with the antioxidants to enhance their protective action.

Remember, it's a basic tenet of the Nashville Diet to pack your cells with concentrated nutrients that are as close as possible to their natural context.

MASTERS OF METABOLISM

You can think of your "metabolism" as simply the overall body process that absorbs and uses nutrients from food as it eliminates what's left over—waste, or toxins. A humming, efficient metabolism—not calorie deprivation—is the key to fat loss in the Nashville Diet.

If you're overweight, your metabolism is not humming or efficient. It's compromised. Nutraplenishing improves your metabolism in several ways. First, it provides the nutrients that the cells need to carry out the metabolic processes. The resulting decrease in food cravings mean fewer calories will be consumed and then stored as fat. Then your improved fat-to-muscle ratio further enhances your metabolic efficiency. Next thing you know, you're a lean, mean, fat-burning machine.

All of the nutrients you'll be packing help your metabolism. But the special purpose of the nutrients in this Masters of Metabolism category is to kick-start the process, and then regularly give it a boost to keep it running smoothly on all cylinders.

Some do this because they're thermogenic, meaning they provide heat. In a sense, they rig your metabolic system's thermostat to improve its performance. Some stimulate your central nervous system, which can increase your metabolic rate. And some assist long-term metabolic health by protecting and detoxifying your liver.

And they all do it naturally. Keep in mind that these nutraceuticals are natural plant substances rich in phytochemicals. So they'll also provide antioxidant, anti-inflammatory, and antibacterial protection.

Many of the supplements in this category deliver caffeine in its natural context. This is part of their power. However, it means you'll have to stop drinking coffee or tea while you're nutraplenishing with these products. The extra caffeine can make you uncomfortable and is not good or healthy. Moreover, caffeine from coffee will diminish the benefits of these supplements. As I'll explain in the next chapter, you'll be rotating your intake of many of these metabolism masters to optimally mete out their effects. Rotation also ensures that you'll be getting the benefits with safe amounts of caffeine. Extra caffeine from coffee or tea will upset the necessary balance.

As with all nutraceuticals, you should consult your doctor before supplementing with these metabolism boosters. For some people, any caffeine at all is not a good idea.

ENERGIZERS

These nutraceuticals naturally increase your alertness, your energy, and, most importantly for our fat-loss mission, your metabolism.

Green tea. What you may enjoy occasionally as a hot tea with Japanese cuisine is even more beneficial as a concentrated powdered extract. Caffeine is just one of the several phytochemicals known as xanthines that are in green tea. They boost your metabolism by stimulating your central nervous system.

Green tea is also loaded with polyphenols, antioxidant phytochemicals that inhibit tumor production and fend off bacteria.

Guarana. Guarana is a berry from Venezuela and northern Brazil that's been used to make a soft drink that's gaining popularity in our country. What you want, though, is the concentrated powder in capsules. The main constituent is guaranine, which is essentially the same as caffeine. But it's also rich in saponins and tannins, two other phytochemicals that enhance mental activity and combat drowsiness. Guarana and green tea work together to improve your metabolism through stimulation of your central nervous system.

Yerba maté. Yerba maté is another South American plant that's rich in xanthines, most notably mateine. Mateine stimulates your central nervous system, boosting metabolism. But it acts differently from caffeine. For example, it improves sleep quality rather than combating drowsiness. So yerba maté will serve to balance the action of green tea and guarana.

Ginseng. You need two different ginsengs—Panax ginseng and Siberian ginseng. They're actually not related botanically, but they work together to increase energy. The metabolism boost from these ginsengs is minimal but, like yerba maté, they balance the effect of the caffeine in green tea and guarana. That balancing not only reduces the potential side effects of the caffeine (like irritability and anxiety), but also helps facilitate the rotation schedule you'll be using to reap the maximum benefits from your metabolism-boosting nutrients.

Ginsengs are also well known for health benefits above and beyond their role in our metabolism-boosting regimen. They protect against liver toxins, lower cholesterol, enhance your stress tolerance, and boost your immune and hormonal systems.

Ginseng is so popular that the market's flooded with inferior products that either use low-grade ginseng roots or otherwise lack the active ingredients. In the case of Panax ginseng, look for a product that promises at least 5 percent of the main active ingredient, ginsenoside. For Siberian ginseng (*Eleutherococcus senticosus*), you'll need to talk with an honest and knowledgeable store manager or other expert to make sure you're getting potent ginseng.

Alpha-lipoic acid (ALA). Recent studies out of the University of California, Berkeley, have pointed to remarkable antiaging powers in this supplement, with one researcher remarking that old rats fed alpha-lipoic acid "got up and did the macarena."

It's believed that ALA revives memory, enhances energy, and improves cellular functioning. Why such powers? It's a strong antioxidant that's naturally produced in the energy-generating areas of your cells, called the mitochondria. It's also one of the few antioxidants that can penetrate the mitochondria from the outside, which explains why supplementing with ALA will boost your energy and your metabolism along with it.

Liver Tonics

Sound liver function is absolutely essential for your health. Anything your body digests passes through the liver to be cleared of toxins before entering the bloodstream. A poorly functioning liver will result in, among many other things, a faltering body metabolism. That in turn negatively affects your vigor, your alertness, and your ability to shed excess body fat.

Because they're liver tonics (meaning they protect and mend your liver) the following nutrients will help prevent those problems.

Curcumin. Curcumin is in the Indian spice turmeric. It's what makes curry yellow. Curcumin's active phytochemicals, called curcuminoids, are antioxidants and anti-inflammatories. It's a liver tonic, but it's also much more. Recent research points to the age-old use of curcumin in central India as the reason why the elderly there suffer far less Alzheimer's disease than their Western counterparts.

Using turmeric as a spice in your food is recommended. But to get the effects you need, curcumin capsules need to be part of your nutra-plenishing line-up.

Dandelion. The greens of the dandelion are gaining some popularity as a healthy salad ingredient. For your nutraplenishing, however, you'll be taking capsules of the powdered root. Dandelion's health benefits are so varied that I could have included it in just about any category in this chapter. It aides digestion by helping the liver release bile, an important digestive juice. It promotes hormone balance by aiding the removal of excess estrogen. And it assists in the removal of toxins from the body. And, of course, it's an excellent general liver tonic.

Milk thistle. The main active ingredient in milk thistle capsules is silymarin, which has a well-documented liver-enhancing function. Milk thistle benefits your liver in two ways. One, it strengthens the liver cell membranes, preventing toxins from penetrating. Two, it actually stimulates the growth of new liver cells. In so doing, it inhibits liver damage from chemicals, drugs, alcohol, and viruses.

N-Acetyl-L-cysteine. Usually abbreviated NAC, this is the delivery form of the liver-protective amino acid L-cysteine. NAC contributes to the creation of the glutathione protein, a powerful antioxidant and detoxifier that plays a big role in the health of your liver. You'll easily find NAC capsules at your health food store. But don't confuse it with N-acetyl-L-carnitine.

HORMONE HELPERS

Hormones are your body's internal chemical messengers. Released by glands through the bloodstream, they control the function of most cells and tissues.

One of the harmful results of nutrient depletion is hormonal imbalance. But to the rescue come the nutraceuticals I'm introducing to you here. Because they balance your hormonal system, they'll further satisfy your body's demands for nutrients, which is the main goal of nutraplenishing.

Your hormone helpers consist of two minerals that act as hormone balancers, two potent herbs that offer hormone-like activity, an actual hormone provider (from a source that might surprise you), and four amino acids.

What's important to keep in mind with these nutraceuticals is that their benefits go well beyond hormone balancing. When your endocrine (hormonal) system is operating at full strength, your immune system also benefits. What's more, your metabolism increases its efficiency, helping you build lean muscle mass and lose fat—the cornerstone of the Nashville Diet.

MINERALS FOR HORMONE MODULATION

You'll hear the term "hormone modulation" referring to artificial hormone replacement, but that's not what we're talking about here. What we're going for is improving your natural hormonal balance by boosting production and distribution. Supplementation with these two minerals will do that, and a lot more.

Chromium. Chromium is a key mineral in nutraplenishing. Its most outstanding benefit is optimizing the activity of insulin, the hormone that directs the way your cells process the sugars and fat from digested food. When insulin is out of balance, accumulated body fat can result, not to mention diabetes and heart disease. That should give you a pretty good idea of the importance of chromium for your vibrant health and fat-loss goals!

There's more, though. Chromium can be ergogenic, meaning it increases muscle mass as it reduces body fat. It helps reduce total cholesterol and triglycerides, as well as inflammation—three benefits that lower your risk for cardiovascular disease. And it stimulates the immune system by increasing the output of invader-fighters called immunoglobulins.

Though chromium is found in grains and meat, it's hard to get in your diet. Even Fregetables aren't sufficient sources of chromium. So chromium's going to be something of an exception in your nutraplenishing scheme, in that you'll be taking it in a form that requires a "delivery molecule" rather than as it occurs naturally in food. But here's the good news: The form we'll be using, called chromium picolinate, turns out to be an excellent source of chromium, allowing for easy absorption. And it's easy to find at health food stores.

Boron. Boron is another nutrient you'll be taking via a delivery molecule, in this case boron citrate. It's found in fruits and vegetables, but the soil is so often poor in boron that even the best diets can't ensure adequate boron intake. (So what else is new?) Boron's a trace mineral that your body needs in very small amounts. But it *does* need those amounts, and the surest way to get boron is by taking it as a separate supplement.

Studies tell us that boron influences your body's hormonal responses to vitamin D, calcium, and magnesium. It turns out that boron plays a key role in calcium metabolism, and therefore helps prevent osteoporosis and osteoarthritis. Boron also helps maintain adequate blood levels of estradiol (an important kind of estrogen) and testosterone. Hence an adequate supply of boron in the body is thought to have an antiaging effect and even to give a youthful, vibrant appearance.

HERBS FOR HORMONE-LIKE ACTIVITY

One of the many ill effects of modern food processing is that it leads to an insufficient intake of plant hormones called phytosterols. So we're going to include on our nutraceutical menu two incredible herbs that are superb sources of phytosterols.

Wild yam root. The wild yam plant (*Dioscorea villosa*) found in the southern United States and parts of Canada is so rich in phytosterols that it's been recommended as a natural alternative for estrogen replacement therapy. The main nutrient involved is an estrogenic compound called diosgenin that was used in the first commercial production of estrogen, progesterone, and other sex hormones. Diosgenin has been shown to stimulate mammary tissue growth.

Wild yam has been used therapeutically to relieve bilious colic and nausea in pregnant women. But you'll be taking the powdered root (or rhizome) in capsule form daily to help restore hormonal imbalances, which can ease premenstrual syndrome (PMS) and menopause symptoms. The phytosterols in wild yam also have immune-modulating capability, enhancing the production of T cells, which are key commanding officers in your immune system's defensive army.

Mexican sarsaparilla. Like wild yam, sarsaparilla (*Smilax medica*) delivers phytosterols, so it provides hormonal activity. Also like wild yam, it contains saponins, which are claimed to be tonics, or blood purifiers.

A HORMONE PROVIDER

The product you're looking for here is bovine orchic substance. You might see it in health food stores as just "orchic." I recommend it for women for this reason: It stimulates the production of the female hormone progesterone and the small amount of the male hormone testosterone that women need to create lean muscle mass. Remember, muscle mass doesn't mean bulky or muscle-bound; it refers to the kind of tissue you want instead of body fat.

Orchic substance doesn't actually supply testosterone to your body. (If it did, I wouldn't recommend it.) Instead, it's a hormone helper, providing your body with the raw material it needs to produce testosterone when it's called for.

Where does bovine orchic substance come from? From male calves. What part? Let's just say the two parts you'd expect to have something to do with testosterone production. I'll spare you more specific details, but if you grew up on a Texas ranch, like I did, you may have been treated to "calf fries" from time to time. At these dinners you ingested your share of orchic substance, with a knife and fork. With nutraplenishing, you'll just swallow a capsule.

Amino Acids

Amino acids, alone or in combination, can have specific physiological effects similar to hormones, thus transcending their role as the basic building blocks of protein. The four that I'm recommending are an important part of your nutraplenishing strategy. Though they support the immune function and have anti-inflammatory activity, I'm including these amino acid supplements as "hormone helpers" because their hormone-like activity helps your body cope better with stress. And many of my clients have reported that this combination of amino acids helped with their hormone-related depression and/or PMS symptoms.

You might find all four of these amino acids together in a blend. However, make sure that they're present in sufficient amounts (we'll get into your dosages in the next chapter). And there shouldn't be too many other amino acids in the blend, since many amino acids compete for the same receptor sites and can neutralize each other.

Arginine. Arginine boosts the release of several hormones, including prolactin and growth hormone (somatotropin) from the pituitary, and insulin and glucagon from the pancreas. It improves the immune system by regulating the thymus gland's production of certain T cells. It helps create lean muscle mass, and it plays a role in liver health.

Arginine is also thought to improve circulation and reduce overall cholesterol. It's often used today to improve sexual health in men and women—a benefit that could be the result of its capacity to help create nitric oxide in the body.

You'll also see it labeled L-arginine. Buy it in the form of L-arginine monohydrochloride.

Lysine. Recently, it's been found that lysine enhances your calcium balance by helping with calcium absorption and blunting its release in the urine. That has important implications for the health of your bones. Lysine is best known as an antiviral agent that effectively fights recurrence of the herpes simplex virus.

You'll also see it as L-lysine, and in the form of L-lysine monohydrochloride.

Glycine. Glycine makes up a third of the amino acid content in collagen, essential for construction and repair of skin, tendons, and other connective tissue.

It also works together with arginine and lysine to regulate the release of growth hormone, or somatotropin.

Glutamine. Glutamine is the most highly concentrated amino acid in the blood, but glutamine supplementation is still beneficial. Its uses in the body are many, including fueling the muscles during stress. Glutamine fits right in with our nutraplenishing goals, because its recruitment in abundant amounts by the gastrointestinal tract decreases hunger cravings.

DETOX DELIGHTS

Your last category of nutraceuticals lays the foundation for your ongoing detoxification efforts by getting your digestive system functioning in fine form. If you're overweight, I guarantee you that you're not digesting food and eliminating waste the way you should be. Nutraplenishing with the supplements I'm about to describe is your first and biggest step toward resurrecting a digestive system that can really head 'em up and move 'em out.

The digestive system starts at your mouth and salivary glands and runs down through your esophagus, stomach, and other digestive organs and on through your intestines. When any part of this intricate system is out of balance as a consequence of undernourishment of the cells, bowel elimination is slowed and unwanted toxins are absorbed without being purged. Any number of unpleasant symptoms can arise—anorexia, dyspepsia, diarrhea, constipation, gastritis, irritable bowel syndrome, to name just a few.

What's more, there's a domino effect, because toxic buildup and poor nutrient absorption can easily cause problems with your immune and cardiovascular systems.

Your Detox Delights support a well-functioning digestive system in many ways, including enhancing the secretion of digestive juices, restoring the population of friendly bacteria in the gut, delivering fiber to keep things moving through, and enriching the supply of digestive enzymes.

And as you'll see in Part Two, all of this leads not just to better health, but also to one of the components of better health that you're most interested in—fat loss

SECRETION AIDS

Dyspepsia is a common syndrome of poor digestion. It refers to bloating, flatulence, and abdominal discomfort because of deficient secretion of gastric juice from the stomach, bile from the gallbladder, and pancreatic juice from the pancreas, as well as production of bile by the liver. You'll be taking in capsulated form two herbs that work together synergistically to get those juices flowing, often eliminating those dyspepsia symptoms as the herbs improve your digestion.

Artichoke. Clinical studies have shown that moderate amounts of concentrated extract from the leaves of the artichoke *(Cynara scolymus)*

do wonders for dyspeptic complaints, as well as for bloating and nausea. The main active component in artichoke, the phytochemical cynarin, works to improve bile secretion and liver function.

Rosemary. You may think of rosemary as nothing more than a flavor in your spice cabinet. (Isn't it interesting how the instinctive desire to have a particular taste or flavor is actually our body's cry for certain nutrients? Isn't God amazing in His attention to detail?) But as a concentrated nutraceutical rich in antioxidant flavonoids, rosemary *(Rosmarinus officinalis)*is a powerful digestion aid and detoxifier.

It works with artichoke to relieve ongoing stomach discomfort by turning up the flow of digestive juices. But it's also been shown to possess anti-inflammatory activity, meaning it may also relieve the kind of inflammations in the digestive tract that lead to ulcers.

Rosemary also has immune system benefits. The same constituents in its oil that create its aromatic appeal also exhibit antibacterial and antifungal properties. It's also good for your circulatory system because it appears to strengthen capillaries.

Fiber Sources

What's the most prevalent adverse condition of the digestive system in our times? Constipation. (Somehow, I think you knew that!)

But constipation might be more prevalent than you thought. If the frequency of your bowel movements is less than once a day, you're probably constipated. And the resulting slowness in waste elimination means more unwanted toxins are being absorbed into your circulatory system, and more fat cells accumulate.

The reason there's so much chronic constipation will be familiar to you by now: an undernourishing diet of depleted food, specifically, in this case, processed food from which fibers have been refined out.

Fiber adds bulk to the stool, which in turn presses on the colon wall, triggering muscle contractions and the urge to defecate.

When you improve your eating habits (which you will) and start drinking more water (which you also will), things will improve. But the first order of business is to pack in natural fiber to help you turn the corner. Here's what you'll do that with:

Fenugreek. Fenugreek is one of those ancient herbs that's been used medicinally since Egyptian times. Our interest in it is based on its high content of galactomannan, a highly effective soluble fiber. Galactomannan also has been shown to help maintain healthy blood sugar levels while lowering insulin response to meals. That means it contributes to optimal metabolism, which is so important for fat loss.

At your health food store, look for the powdered seed of fenugreek (*Trigonella foenum*) in capsules.

Flaxseed. The lignan and cellulose in flaxseed provides more fiber that works synergistically with fenugreek to lower cholesterol levels, control blood glucose, and improve gastrointestinal function. Flaxseed fiber is commonly used to treat chronic constipation and colon problems. Again, look for the powdered seed of flaxseed *(Linum usitatissimum)* in capsules.

Rice bran. Rice bran comes in two basic forms, the powdered bran or the bran in oil form. It is one of the richest sources of vitamins, minerals, and antioxidants found in nature. Rice bran and germ from all-natural processes capture the nutritional power of the planet's most significant and abundant food.

Rice bran oil (RBO) contains powerful antioxidants that may reduce cholesterol, promote heart health, and reduce the risk of cancer. The benefits of RBO for health and beautiful skin and hair have been known in Asia, especially Japan, for many generations. RBO is a primary component of cosmetics in Japan, where it is believed to greatly enhance the beauty of skin and hair. RBO applications are a regular part of beauty treatments in the best salons in Japan. Many persons with dry or scaly skin find marked improvement within a week of taking one to two tablespoons of RBO daily. Applying it externally to you hair adds body and a healthful luster. Recent research has confirmed that RBO is one of the best sources of tocotrienol, an antioxidant that may be many times more powerful and effective than vitamin E.

DIGESTIVE ENZYMES

Enzymes are proteins that do things. One of the things they do is trigger the chemical reactions that digest food and break down toxins. Unfortunately, whatever enzymes in food survive depleted soils, green harvesting, and industrial processing are lost during cooking. So your body has to tap its own enzyme reserves, which includes your immune system. That's how enzyme depletion puts a strain on your immune system as well as your gastrointestinal (digestive) system.

The solution is to include digestive enzymes in your nutraplenishing. The benefits of enzyme supplementation go beyond better digestion. Your immune system will also be helped, as well as your blood sugar levels and overall cholesterol count.

Health food stores offer a potpourri of digestive enzyme blends. The general category of enzymes you want is known as the hydrolases or the hydrolytic digestive enzymes. The types of hydrolases to look for are proteases, lipases, and amylases. Also look for cellulase, a sub-type of amylase enzyme that your body does not manufacture itself. Cellulase helps you digest raw food and helps your system deal with fungi and yeast.

A PROBIOTIC

The final tool in your Detox Delight kit is a single probiotic—that is, beneficial microorganism—known as *Lactobacillus sporogenes*. This probiotic is able to survive the gastric juices of your stomach and end up in your intestine, where it produces short-chain fatty acids, lactic acids, and butyric acids. Those chemicals create an environment favoring the growth conditions of friendly bacteria responsible for healthy digestion and detoxification of harmful waste.

BEFORE YOU BUY

Now you've been introduced to the remarkable nutraceuticals that will replenish your long-suffering, nutrient-depleted cells. But don't run out to buy them just yet. I've told you what to nutraplenish with. But I haven't told you how much of it to take, or how often. In the next chapter, I'm going to lay out your nutraplenishing plan. I'll show you the roadmap for the first part of your journey from fat to lean.

secrets to successful supplementation

you now have your line-up of the nutrient supplements that will take you from fat to lean. This combination of nutraceuticals that make up the Nashville Diet nutraplenishing plan was formulated with one goal in mind. That goal is to restore your cellular health and encourage the best eating habits by providing your body with the most important nutritional components missing from even the best of diets.

Out of the literally hundreds of nutrients lacking in our food supply, the nutraceuticals selected for this comprehensive nutritional program are the result of extensive research. More importantly, they're the product of direct, hands-on experience—by me, my colleagues, and countless clients who came to me with the same weight and energy problems that you're experiencing now. We've all taken these supplements and will continue to take them. We know they work.

You may be wondering: Why these supplements and not the seemingly thousands of others that fill the shelves? That's an excellent question, because there really are a lot more nutrient supplements out there that can do you plenty of good. But nobody can take them all, nor should they.

So I made some roster cuts (to use a sports metaphor) to come up with the best team possible.

A big reason this particular collection of supplements is so effective for fat loss is the synergistic effect of the combinations. What that means, basically, is that these nutrients work together so well that they actually enhance each other's benefits. It's like two plus two equaling ten.

Again, the capsules you'll be taking every day contain food, not medicine. But it's food in a special, concentrated form that delivers nutrients for the cells. So while most people think of a diet as a series of instructions for what foods to choose and how much of them to eat, the Nashville Diet is all about what nutrient supplements to choose and how much of them to take. You've learned what they are. Now let's see how much to take.

MAPPING YOUR FAT-TO-LEAN COURSE

Everybody is different. So is every body. No two will respond alike to the nourishing effects of the nutrients in the Nashville Diet. Although the nutraplenishing regimen I've developed is appropriate for anybody who wants to lose fat by improving internal health, everyone should progress at her or his own pace.

How do you know what your pace is? Your best guide is your own body.

Listen to it. Lower your doses when your body seems to be reacting uncomfortably to a certain nutrient group. On the other hand, if you're not feeling more energy and decreased food cravings in a fairly short time, your doses may be too low or the quality of the supplements you're taking may not be up to par. Adjust accordingly. Otherwise, move forward along the schedule I'll be giving you shortly.

As important as this self-monitoring is, even the most diligent body-listeners need a starting point. Nourishing your cells with these powerful nutrients represents a radical change from what your body is used to. Few folks can just dive into the deep end. Some need to wade in slowly. Others might just stick in a toe or two to get started. How do you know where to begin?

The determining factor is your overall health. For my clinical practice I developed a method for measuring that overall health. It's called the

Vibrant Health Index, or VHI, and you use it to establish your body's health "baseline," and then as an objective means for measuring improvements as you follow the Nashville Diet. Instead of using a shot-in-the-dark approach to nutraplenishing, knowing your current Vibrant Health Index score helps you pinpoint which nutrients to take, how much of each, and how to adjust them for maximum benefit.

I'm going to show you an easy way to find your Vibrant Health Index score. Then I will show you how to use that number to fine-tune your nutraplenishing regimen (and later to detoxify your cells). From now on, your health status will have a number. As that number gets higher over the coming weeks (and it will get higher if you follow the program) you'll be that much closer to achieving the vibrant health you deserve.

WHAT IS THIS THING CALLED "VIBRANT HEALTH"?

You may be wondering what I mean when I talk about "vibrant health" so much. When you have all of your vibrant health, you have the strength, energy, happy attitude, and lean, muscular body of a fit teenager—but with the maturity, experience, and intelligence of a person your age.

Impossible, you say? It may seem like it when you're feeling sick, fat, lazy, and discouraged.

But it's not impossible because vibrant health is your body's preferred state. It's where your body would be if your cells were fully nourished, detoxified, and functioning as they're supposed to. Your Vibrant Health Index score tells you how close you are to that natural ideal.

The VHI test you'll be taking regularly condenses years of research and clinical practice into thirty-three questions that measure how you feel, which is where the rubber hits the road. After all, how you look is a direct result of how you feel. And if you're going to look and feel good it will be from the inside out. The pleasing glow and trim figure that I see in clients who have graduated from my program are merely outward signs of their greatly improved inner health.

For the purposes of nutraplenishing and cleansing toxins from your systems, the VHI approach gives you a more valuable picture than the typical urine or blood tests that a physician might use for diagnostic purposes. Blood tests can be deceptive because our body's homeostasis mechanism gives top priority to balancing the supply of all life-sustaining nutrients in the blood supply, making your blood "look" fine. Since our blood feeds and balances our entire body, it gets whatever it needs, regardless of the cost. The example I gave earlier about how your body uses calcium is a perfect illustration. A blood test might indicate perfectly acceptable calcium levels in your bloodstream, with no indication that your body is actually starved for the stuff, and stealing it from your bones.

Your Vibrant Health Index Questionnaire

Determine your current Vibrant Health Index by filling out the questionnaire (Appendix A on p. 253). It's a simple matter of giving yourself a score for each question about your health. Usually, you'll score yourself on a scale of 0 to 5, with 5 indicating that a particular health problem is severe or intense, and a 0 meaning no problem exists. To remind you, there will usually be a phrase next to the 5 on the 0–5 scale briefly describing a typical 5 score, and a phrase next to the 0 describing the ideal score. Your answer may lie between, or at either of the extremes. Use your judgment. You know best! A few questions allow for a score higher than 5.

Write your score in the space to the right of each question, in the blank after the word "score." If the phrase "score X 2" appears before the blank, double your score and write the doubled number in the space provided. Unless otherwise indicated, base your answer on your situation today, the day you're taking your VHI.

Don't enter your scores directly in the book. Make several copies of the VHI questionnaire. (You'll find it on p. 253.) If you have access to a computer, and the interest, you can take the Vibrant Health Index online at www.NashvilleDiet.com, where it will calculate your score and provide nutrient recommendations. You'll need to take your VHI weekly for the first two months, or until your VHI gets into the 80s.

After that, it would be a good idea to take the VHI at the first of each month to make sure you'll be staying on the vibrant health track for the rest of your life.

WHAT YOUR VHI SCORE MEANS TO YOU

Now that you've got a number that represents your Vibrant Health Index, you'll want to know how to use it. Again, your VHI score is important for losing weight through nutraplenishing because it helps you determine which nutrients you'll be taking at first, as well as how much of each.

Basically, the score is like grading in school. Over 90 is the best, an excellent grade, an "A." Under 60 means you're "failing" to enjoy your vibrant health and you've got lots of work to do. But there's a big difference between your VHI and an academic grade. Your VHI score, even if it's low, in no way reflects your achievement, or your ability, or your effort level. It's simply a marker of your current state of health and energy as it applies to your fat-loss/energy-increase strategies. Believe me, a lot of my clients crawl in with VHIs lower than the Tennessee temperature in January. But they all walk out with the tools to keep their vibrant health for a lifetime. So don't be discouraged if your VHI is low, you're the one we can help the most. Your VHI score is simply validating what you already knew—that you want more energy and less fat. Now let's take a more detailed look at what these numbers tell you about your health and your nutraplenishing schedule.

If Your VHI Is Under 60

You are quite sick and undernourished, and probably or quite a bit overweight. You're also very toxic, so you'll want to pay special attention to Part Two of this book. You are most likely under a doctor's care and should continue to be as you follow the Nashville Diet. You surely didn't get this way overnight, so it will take some time to get out of the jungle. (It took me two years to come all the way back.) But you can do it. And you're not alone.

Because you're so toxic, you'll have to begin your nutraplenishing very slowly so you don't stir up too many toxins at once. You must introduce one nutrient group at a time using a single, minimum dose of each individual nutrient. Gauge how you feel for several days with one nutrient group before adding the next. Start with the Immune Boosters, then add the Fregetables, then the Hormone Helpers. Don't take any of the Masters of Metabolism or Detox Delights until your VHI is in the 70s.

If Your VHI Is in the 60s

You know that you're not very healthy. You have significant problems with undernourishment and toxicity. Your weight is probably an issue, as is your energy level. It's also likely that you're taking a number of medications. Many people in this VHI range have tried a lot of avenues to health and fat loss with little lasting success. You may be discouraged and ready to give up. *Don't!* You're precisely the kind of person that nutraplenishing helps the most.

You'll need to go slow with your nutrient regimen, starting with a single daily dose of Immune Boosters, Fregetables, and Hormone Helpers. You'll have to hold off on the Masters of Metabolism and the Detox Delights until your VHI hits 70, but you'll be able to double your dosages of the nutrients you do take before that if you show some improvement, at least a 5-point increase on the VHI. Move up in dosage one nutrient group at a time. Pay attention to the VHI requirements for each nutrient group when you get to the dosage recommendations below.

If Your VHI Is in the 70s

You're in average health, which isn't good enough. You're still toxic, malnourished, and probably overweight. A lot of clients at this VHI level feel okay some of the time, but go down quickly with any illness or setback. You're in a good position to learn to listen to your body and get the most out of nutraplenishing. You're ahead of a lot of people, so make up your mind to go forward and you will succeed. Your VHI is high enough to take all the nutrient groups, though you should phase-in the Detox Delights last. Your dosages will be limited until you hit 80; check the VHI requirements for each nutrient group below.

If Your VHI Is in the 80s

Congratulations! You're in good condition, probably less toxic than most (though by no means toxin-free), and not too far from excellent health. You still have some work to do, though. You surely need to lose body fat and you may still be craving some foods, such as salt, red meat, alcohol, sweets, caffeine, or dairy.

You're poised to enjoy the full benefits of nutraplenishing and reach your ideal weight. You can phase in all of the nutrient groups from the beginning, with just a few limitations from the VHI requirements given in each group's dosage information below.

If Your VHI Is in the 90s

You are truly special. You pretty much have all of your vibrant health. You're energetic, productive, happy, and able to leap tall buildings in a single bound. Chances are you've reached this level after nutraplenishing for some months; rare is the newcomer with a VHI in the 90s. You may still have some fat to get rid of, though, so keep taking your nutrients so you'll stay nourished and eat healthy.

Onward and Upward

Unless your VHI is in the upper 90s, your ongoing goal is to get that number higher by following your nutraplenishing regimen faithfully, in addition to the detoxification strategies and healthy eating advice I'll be sharing with you later. Your VHI will be a constant reminder that your fat-loss and vibrant health goals are intimately intertwined.

Now it's time to put your VHI to use by applying it to a nutraplenishing regimen—that is, how much to take of which nutrients, and how often.

YOUR NUTRAPLENISHING REGIMEN

Even though your nutrient supplements are simply concentrated food, it's still absolutely vital to follow a carefully prepared plan for introducing them to your body. You've been without sufficient supplies of these nutrients for so long that their sudden reintroduction, as beneficial as it is, will be a radical change that your body needs to adjust to gradually.

The most compelling reason for progressing slowly toward your eventual full nutraplenishing regimen has to do with the toxins nesting in fat cells throughout your body. Because these health-harming toxins contribute to your weight problem, the Nashville Diet is designed to eliminate them.

You'll learn all about this important part of the program in the next three chapters. For now, be aware that even the very first nutrient supplement you take starts the process of pulling those toxins out of your cells. That's a good thing, of course, but it can be an uncomfortable thing, too, as you "stir up" long-hidden toxins.

The regimen below is designed to deliver the maximum health and fat-loss benefits with a minimum of "toxic symptoms." *Please follow it.*

SOME BASIC GUIDELINES . . .

Now, before we get into the details, here are some guidelines to help you understand how your supplementation schedule will work:

- Organize your supplements by the five nutrient categories—Immune Boosters, Fregetables, Masters of Metabolism, Hormone Helpers, and Detox Delights. That's the way the regimen below is presented. For one thing, it's a lot easier to keep track of five categories than thirty-plus individual nutrients. More important, though, is that you'll always be taking all of the nutrients in any one category at the same time. For that reason, it's a good idea to actually store your supplements by category, so when it comes time to take, say, your Hormone Helpers, they'll all be right there together.

- ☐ Use the "one dose" figure of each nutrient as your guide. The regimen below tells you what a single dose is for each nutrient—the minimum amount of that nutrient you'd take at a time. Remember, each nutrient has its own single dose, so the single dose will vary from nutrient to nutrient, even within the same category.

- ☐ When the schedule tells you to take two doses of a category, that means double the dosage of every nutrient within that category.

- ☐ Nutrient supplements are usually measured in milligrams, which is often abbreviated "mg." A milligram is one-thousandth of a gram. There are about 28 grams in an ounce. Occasionally, a nutrient will be measured in micrograms (mcg), a measurement even smaller than a milligram (mg). The number of milligrams or micrograms of any nutrient in a capsule should be clearly marked on the bottle it comes in.

- ☐ Make sure the amount of the nutrient in the actual capsule corresponds to the dosage the schedule tells you to take. For example, the aloe vera product you buy may consist of 50-milligram capsules. Since our single dose of aloe vera is 100 milligrams, you need two capsules for a single dose.

- ☐ You may run into problems if the product's capsules contain more of the nutrient than our single dose. Don't try to take apart the capsule and measure out the right amount. Instead, look for products with capsule dosages that correspond to or are less than our dosages. If the dosages are off by a small percentage, that's okay. For example, if you need a single dose of wild yam root at 120 milligrams, but you can only find 50-milligram capsules, your single dose will have to be either 100 milligrams or 150 milligrams.

☐ "Pyramid-in" your full regimen by introducing one nutrient category at a time. Phase them in this order: Immune Boosters, Fregetables, Hormone Helpers, Masters
of Metabolism, Detox Delights. By introducing only one
new category at a time, you're better able to monitor your
body's response to each.

☐ The single dose is often a minimum that you will build on
as your body adjusts. In other words, you'll start with whatever dosage is recommended according to your VHI and
then work your way up to your full regimen. But don't increase your dosage for more than one category at a time.
Again, that helps you keep track of the effects of any one
dosage increase, and at the same time gives your body
time to adjust and remove the toxins that are released by
this process.

☐ Unless otherwise indicated, take your capsules in the
morning. If you take more than one dose, split them between morning and lunchtime.

☐ From day one, keep a day-by-day chart of your nutrient
intake. Arrange it any way you like, but you should be
able to tell at a glance what dosages you've taken in the
past, what you're scheduled to take today, and what
dosage increases are planned for the future (though you
may not always know the exact date of those future
increases).

Are you ready to start? Good!

Here's your nutraplenishing regimen, category by category:

IMMUNE BOOSTERS

If you're starting your nutraplenishing with just one category of supplements, this is the one to start with. It includes aloe vera, arabinogalactan,

and MSM. Don't forget that your aloe vera *absolutely* must be in a 200:1 concentration, or it won't provide the desired benefits.

IMMUNE BOOSTERS SINGLE DOSE

NUTRIENT	DOSE
ALOE VERA.	100 MG
AG	100 MG
MSM	50 MG

Immune Boosters Dosage Recommendations

VHI 70s: Take two doses of this combination daily from the first day. *Optional*: Move up to three daily doses after the first week.

VHI 60s: Take only one dose to begin with. Move up to two a day after a week if you've already phased in the Fregetables and Hormone Helpers, and your VHI hasn't dropped.

VHI 50s: Start with one dose a day. Monitor carefully how you feel each day. Move up to two doses after you have phased in Fregetables and Hormone Helpers, but only if your VHI has risen 5 points.

FREGETABLES

Try to find the concentrated cruciferous vegetables in blends that include all four of my recommended nutrients (it can include some others). And make sure it's the highest quality product. If it is, you shouldn't have to worry about allergic reactions to the powdered vegetable concentrates, even if you're prone to allergies. Most of the time any allergic reaction with vegetable capsules is due to the residue of chemicals from pesticides and fertilizers, not the plant material itself.

FREGETABLES SINGLE DOSE :   500—600 MG

To reach that total, you have some leeway. First, break the nutrients in this category into three categories:

1. The cruciferous vegetables (broccoli, Brussels sprouts, cabbage, kale).
2. Papaya and pineapple.
3. Tomato, carrot, and blueberry (and/or elderberry).

Now, put together a combination of all the nutrients that totals 500 – 600 mg, and that's one dose. The lion's share should go to the cruciferous group, with the tomato/carrot/blueberry group in second place. The papaya and pineapple will combine for less than 50 mg. Fregetables will be the second nutrient category you'll be taking, phasing it in after you start the Immune Boosters

Fregetables Dosage Recommendations

VHI 80s. Take two to four doses daily from the beginning.

VHI 70s. Take up to three per doses per day.

VHI 60s. Take up to two doses per day.

VHI 50s. Take one dose per day, as second step after the one week of one dose of the Immune Boosters.

HORMONE HELPERS

This is the third category of nutrients for you to start taking. It includes amino acids, which need to be taken on an empty stomach for best absorption. Therefore, so you can keep track of what you're taking more easily, take all your Hormone Helpers before breakfast in the morning. The four recommended amino acids are arginine, lysine, glycine, and glutamine. Look for them in a blend.

HORMONE HELPERS SINGLE DOSE

NUTRIENT	DOSE
CHROMIUM	95 MICROGRAMS
BORON	1 MG
MEXICAN SARSAPARILLA	100 MG
WILD YAM ROOT	120 MG

NUTRIENT	DOSE
ORCHIC SUBSTANCE	200 MG
AMINO ACIDS COMBINED	500–700 MG

Hormone Helpers Dosage Recommendations

VHI 80s. Start with two daily doses and build up to four daily doses.

VHI 70s. Start with one dose a day, and add a second dose after one week. Build up to four daily doses.

VHI 60s. Start with one dose per day and add a second dose after a week if you respond well to the first one.

VHI 50s. Before beginning the Hormone Helpers you must have a VHI of at least 60. Take the Immune Booster and Fregetables, and work your way up to two of each dose per day and stay there until your VHI is at least 60, then at that time take one-half of the listed dose. Take this regimen until your VHI is in the 70s, at which time you can begin to add Masters of Metabolism.

MASTERS OF METABOLISM

There are some important considerations for this category of nutrients: *Do not take the Masters of Metabolism if*:

- ☐ You are pregnant or nursing.
- ☐ You have an overactive thyroid.
- ☐ You checked any boxes under questions 31 or 32 in your VHI questionnaire, unless you have an okay from your doctor.
- ☐ **Under no circumstances should you consume caffeinated products if you're taking Masters of Metabolism.** You will be getting a beneficial effect from the small amounts of natural caffeine in some of these nutrients. Additional caffeine consumed in inappropriate contexts will negate the benefits. Too much caffeine may increase your heart rate and blood pressure and possibly

cause health problems. Don't drink coffee, tea, soft drinks, or any other caffeinated beverage. Don't eat chocolate.

☐ Take your Masters of Metabolism in the morning just before breakfast. If you take more than one dose, take the second at lunch. Don't take any later in the day.

☐ To keep your metabolism from hitting plateaus—and therefore to maximize the benefits of these nutrients— eliminate the guarana and yerba maté only on three consecutive days of each week. I suggest Friday through Sunday for this adjusted nutrient make-up. Thus, you'll take the full list of Masters of Metabolism nutrients for four days, and the abbreviated version for three.

MASTERS OF METABOLISM SINGLE DOSE

NUTRIENT	DOSE
GUARANA	200 MG
YERBA MATÉ	100 MG
GREEN TEA EXTRACT	200 MG
GINSENG (PANAX)	100 MG
GINSENG (SIBERIAN)	10 MG
CURCUMIN	20 MG
DANDELION	1 MG
MILK THISTLE	150 MG
N-ACETYL-L-CYSTEINE	50 MG
ALPHA-LIPOIC ACID	100 MG

Masters of Metabolism Dosage Recommendations

VHI 70s. After you have been taking the first three nutrient categories, begin with one dose in the morning. After a week, add a second dose at lunch. On Fridays, Saturdays, and Sundays, eliminate the guarana and yerba maté and take the rest of the dose as normal.

VHI 60s or lower. Don't include these Masters of Metabolism in your regimen until your VHI hits 70. Concentrate on the first three nutrient categories instead. They'll build your internal strength as they nourish and cleanse your cells. You'll get there.

DETOX DELIGHTS

These are primarily digestive aids that take the detoxification effects of nutraplenishing to a more intense level. Therefore, phase these in only after your other nutraplenishing categories have been "up and running" for a few weeks.

DETOX DELIGHTS SINGLE DOSE

NUTRIENT	DOSE
FLAXSEED POWDER	500 MG
RICE BRAN POWDER	400 MG
ARTICHOKE EXTRACT	200 MG
ROSEMARY	50 MG
DIGESTIVE ENZYMES	100 MG
PROBIOTIC	250 MG

Detox Delights Dosage Recommendations

VHI 69 or below. Do not take these nutrients until your VHI reaches 70.

VHI 70s. Take one dose in the morning before breakfast. If you feel fine after a day or two, add a second dose before lunch.

YOUR GOAL IS IN SIGHT!

Starting anything new can be overwhelming, especially if it involves keeping track of more than thirty nutrient supplements! So make it easy on yourself by going slow and being patient with yourself. Keep writing down everything you're doing, and if you get confused or lost, don't worry about it. Just back up and start over on that part of the program. Remember, you're not on some gimmicky lose-weight-quick scheme. You're reclaiming your health for a lifetime. It's not a race.

Never let yourself get discouraged. Never forget that just by taking these nutrients, you're delivering health to your body every day. That would be worth the effort even if you never lost a pound. Countless numbers of clients have said this to me. But I would say that most clients become more interested in their vibrant health than "weight loss" by the time they begin to feel like they are actually alive for the first time most can remember.

But you're going to lose plenty of pounds. Let me give you some facts to illustrate just how rich the rewards of nutraplenishing will be for you.

The average client at my clinic is thirty-five to forty-eight years old and arrives with a VHI of 55. She needs to shrink five sizes. She's on two prescription medications (one is usually an antidepressant) and has been sick and/or overweight for at least ten years. And here's the most intriguing part: She's tried at least six other programs already!

The results? They vary, of course, from client to client, though they're always positive. On average, though, a client will shrink two sizes in ninety days after she begins nutraplenishing, and four sizes in six months. She will get off her prescription medications and have a much happier and more productive life thanks to much more balanced moods and a huge increase in energy.

But you don't have to come to my clinic to lose weight on this plan. Just take your VHI, buy high-quality supplements, and put them in your mouth. Follow the regimen you just read and you're on your way! Nothing can stop you.

You're on the right path . . . finally! Now, let's keep moving ahead toward our goal of a trim and energetic, vibrantly healthy you. Next step: A thorough cleansing of every cell in your body.

2

DETOXIFY YOUR SYSTEM

The Problem:
toxins

congratulate yourself! You deserve it!

You've already taken a huge step toward a lean and healthy body. Even if you haven't swallowed a single nutrient capsule yet, you're miles ahead of the vast majority of yo-yo dieters and fad-followers who will always fail until they learn what you now know.

You know (and they don't) that moving from fat to lean is not a matter of *depriving* your body of food but of *providing* your body with the nutrients it needs to function properly. To get lean, your body needs *more*, not *less*. (Not more calories, of course, but more nourishment.)

You also know that your weight problems and health problems are intricately intertwined, and that the only way to lose your excess weight is to regain your vibrant health.

And best of all, you know that a nutraplenishing regimen consisting of a carefully selected army of health-promoting nutraceuticals is the only way available today to provide your cells with the nourishment they need but can't get from our modern, nutrient-depleted food supply.

The nutraplenishing plan I described for you in the last two chapters gives you exactly what you need to satisfy your cells' nutritional needs. Nutritionally satisfied cells don't bombard you with cravings that push you to eat too much of the wrong foods. And they function better, boosting the efficiency of your digestive, immune, and other important systems as they restore your overall vibrant health.

For those reasons, nutraplenishing is the foundation of the Nashville Diet. But it plays another key role as well. It prepares your body for the second essential component of your fat-to-lean program: detoxification. Detoxification simply means ridding your body of accumulated toxins, especially those in your fat cells. Detox is absolutely vital for a healthy fat-loss strategy. You cannot shed excess body fat and keep it off while allowing harmful toxins to maintain year-round residence in your cells. And if you're overweight, you're virtually sure to have dangerous levels of toxins in your system. Yet detox strategies are almost completely ignored by calorie-deprivation regimens and fad diets. That will not be the case with you. By reading this far, you've demonstrated a personal commitment to your own health. I'm going to honor that commitment by using the rest of this chapter and the two chapters that follow to show you exactly what you must do to cleanse your sacred body of these harmful poisons, thereby shrinking your fat cells and restoring your vibrant health.

THE TOXINS WITHIN YOU

Most of us, when we hear the word "toxin," think of a substance that harms our bodies. That's a pretty good working definition. But from your body's point of view, there's more to it.

The body sees *anything* that's not where it should be as toxic. Even the most benign-seeming elements, like air and water, will be treated as toxic if they're out of place in your body's complex architecture.

There's another preconception you may have about toxins that doesn't tell the whole story. We tend to think of toxic damage only as something imposed from the outside—by pollution and chemical poisons and synthetic pharmaceuticals and food additives. And it's certainly true that these "modern" toxins have pushed the toxicity problem over the edge, creating too much illness and (for reasons you'll soon learn) contributing to the obesity epidemic in our society.

But it's also true that your body is waging an ongoing war against harmful toxins *of its own making*. Even if we lived in a pristine environment, our detox systems would still be working full-time to eliminate abundant natural toxins in the body. Most of these are "endotoxins," by-products of necessary chemical reactions taking place in your cells. To pick a simple example, waste products are created as your body breaks down dietary protein for cell building. This waste is toxic—that is, it's out of place, unwanted, and harmful. It must be eliminated.

Especially harmful among these endotoxins are free radicals, the delinquent oxygen molecules you were introduced to as we discussed antioxidant nutrients in Chapter Three. We know that antioxidants minimize the oxidative or rust-like cellular damage from free radicals. But it takes an endless effort to keep those free radicals in check, just as it takes an endless effort to process other waste products out of your body. Even as you read this, the great Detox War is raging within you.

TOXINS, TOXINS, EVERYWHERE

Under the right circumstances, your liver, digestive system, lymphatic system, and other natural detoxifiers are well equipped to hold their own in the Detox War. Unfortunately, the circumstances haven't been right on most of this earth for many decades. The enemy troops have multiplied as the world has become a very toxic place. At the same time, our defenses have weakened, because the nutrient-depleted food supply fails to provide our detox mechanisms with the raw material they need to work right. Our bodies are overwhelmed with toxins. There are toxins in our food supply, our water supply, the air we breathe, the ground we walk on, the buildings we work in, and the homes we live in. No wonder cancer is so rampant in our society! What's more, environmental toxins are a major reason why obesity levels have skyrocketed. Without taking aggressive steps to detoxify our systems, we don't stand a chance. We can't be healthy. And we can't lose weight. Fortunately, we can indeed take those aggressive steps to detoxify ourselves. But before I tell you how, I'm going to tell you why.

TOXINS: ENEMIES OF FAT LOSS

You might find that detoxification is the most challenging component of the Nashville Diet program. But it's also the most rewarding in terms of restoring your vibrant health. At my practice, we often spend much more time with detox strategies than we do with actual food programs. I know you probably still find it hard to believe, but once you establish a consistent nutraplenishing regimen and bring down your toxin levels, eating right is a snap! (Well, maybe not a *snap*, but much easier than you ever imagined if all you've known is calorie-deprivation diets.)

My clients seem to understand intuitively the importance of detox. Remember, most are quite ill as well as overweight, so the notion of ridding the body of accumulated poison strikes one and all as a darn good idea. But what they don't get at first is the connection between detox and weight loss. Sure, they're all for eliminating excess toxins. But what does that have to do with ridding their bodies of excess fat?

The truth is, fat and toxicity are really two aspects of the same problem. That's why detox is such an essential element of the Nashville Diet. And it's another reason why typical commercial diets that fail to mention the problem of toxin accumulation rarely work in the long run.

FAT AND TOXINS: CROWDED CELLMATES

Remember your first basic biology course in high school? You may recall something about entities called fat cells in our bodies. Bad as they sound, these fat-laden cells are actually essential energy-storage units. Since body fat is basically warehoused energy, fat cells in and of themselves are not the problem. When you take in more calories than your body needs to burn as fuel, the excess caloric energy is stored as fat. Keep it up over time, and those fat deposits overaccumulate. That's why the classic weight-loss strategy is to bring things back into balance by consuming fewer calories while burning more calories with exercise. Fewer unused calories mean less unused energy to store as fat. *Voila!*

Alas, life is not so simple. We've already seen how your body constantly demands more food in a desperate attempt to acquire the nutrients it needs to function properly. What it gets, of course, is more calories to store as fat, but still not enough nutrients. As millions of yo-yo dieters have learned, it's next to impossible to eat fewer calories while trillions of cells are insisting that you eat more. That's a problem that leads to excess body fat. (And it's also a problem that we're solving with nutraplenishing!)

But now it's time to consider another complication. The body also stores away toxins that it's not able to immediately process and eliminate. And guess where those toxins get stored, for the most part? That's right— in fat cells. Hiding excess toxins in fat cells is actually another of your body's marvelous lifesaving strategies. That's because those toxins do far less harm in fat cells than in other places, such as your brain tissue, your liver, and your digestive tract.

Unfortunately, a great deal of toxic matter finds its way to those areas, contributing to migraines, liver disease, and digestive tract problems such as irritable bowel syndrome. All things considered, fat cells are better storage units, although getting rid of the toxins once and for all (as you'll learn to do in the next chapter) is the only healthy solution. Now, these fat cells are only supposed to be temporary holding chambers for soon-to-be-processed toxins. But since your body is bombarded by toxins from within and without all day every day, it can't catch up with its toxin-processing chores, hard as it may try. So those old toxins take up long-term residency in your fat cells.

Think about that for a minute. Your problem isn't just excess body fat. Your problem is excess *toxic* body fat. The toxicity of your body fat must be dealt with, because it complicates your fat-to-lean quest in several ways. I'll mention a few:

Toxic fat means more fat. Accumulated toxins increase the volume of fat cells. You may not have *more* fat cells, but the cells you do have are literally plumped up by their toxic content. That's one reason why toxin removal leads to weight loss.

Toxic fat is stubborn. Have you ever noticed that the more work you let pile up, the harder it is to get started on any of it? It's the same with your body's natural detoxification functions. Toxins can clog your system to such a degree that the more toxins that accumulate, the fewer you're able to eliminate.

Toxic fat starts a vicious cycle. I've seen this happen to countless clients. High toxic exposure leads to weight gain and a feeling of exhaustion. In an attempt to compensate, my clients would eat more of the wrong things—sugar, bread, vinegary or pickled foods. Thus their body fat and stored toxins encourage each other.

Toxic fat discourages fat loss. Your body is a vigilant landlord. It *knows* that toxins have moved into your fat cells. It also knows that "burning" those fat cells to extract their energy will release those toxins into your bloodstream, possibly in harmful amounts. Remember, the reason those toxins were hidden away in your fat cells to begin with was to keep them *out* of the bloodstream. So your body tends to "hold on" to toxin-drenched fat cells, frustrating your fat-loss goals.

I'm sure you've got the message by now that toxins are a huge factor affecting both your weight and your overall health. Much as I hate to be the bearer of bad news, it's important that you have an idea of the extent of the problem in today's world. So before we move on to your detoxification strategy, let's look at what I'm really talking about when I say we live in a toxic world.

Don't be discouraged, though. As you read through the list of toxins that most of us live with daily, keep in mind that soon you will be taking steps to deal with the problem and clear the way for significant fat loss. That's an advantage that few would-be dieters even know about.

TOXINS IN OUR ENVIRONMENT

There's probably never been a time in human history when environmental toxins weren't a problem. Carbon monoxide from fire surely bothered cavemen. And of course parasites and microbes were around long before we were. Today, however, we're in a whole new league.

You're no doubt well aware of modern pollutants such as pesticides, contaminated air, second-hand smoke, and chemical waste. Those are certainly major toxic sources, but by no means the only ones. So if, like some of my clients when they first come in, you assume that you're out of toxic danger because you live in a "clean" area far from the bad air and spewing factories of the big city, I'm sorry to report that you're kidding yourself.

The modern world is saturated with toxins. More than two thousand new chemicals are being introduced into our environment each year. And because our lungs and skin are like big sponges in their ability to absorb just about anything that comes near them, we have the perfect "toxin delivery systems" to bring those toxins into our bodies. It doesn't matter that we may have no idea that the toxins are even around. We lap them up anyway.

The truth is that we can never avoid toxins completely. What we can do, though, is be aware of what they are—and where they are—so we can minimize our exposure. Then we can cleanse ourselves of the toxins we've accumulated so our bodies will have a fighting chance to eliminate the toxins we cannot avoid taking in. And that's exactly what you're going to do in the detoxification stage of the Nashville Diet.

Your first step is to recognize something that may surprise you: The toxic threat to your health is mostly an *indoor* problem. The U.S. Environmental Protection Agency (EPA) tells us that the air quality indoors is as much as five times worse than outdoors. What's more, we spend about 90 percent of our time indoors. In other words, we spend most of our time where most of the toxins are. No wonder indoor pollution, according to the EPA, is one of the top environmental threats in the United States.

MOLD: THE MODERN NEMESIS

Several decades ago, it came to light that asbestos, a fire retardant commonly used for insulation, was a dangerous carcinogen easily absorbed by anyone unfortunate enough to be around it. Today, the most insidious indoor toxin is something you may already be familiar with: mold.

Mold is a fungal growth, a very simple micro-organism. Of the many species of mold, several are very toxic. The most common toxic mold types are called aspergillus and stachybotrys, which often take the form of black clumps. It's easy to be exposed to these species, since they send spores into the air and therefore into your lungs. Just as smoke inhalation kills more people than the fire itself, insidious mold spores are what's most damaging about mold.

Respiratory problems such as asthma and frequent colds head the list of illnesses caused by these molds. But there are countless other symptoms, including allergies, ear infections, yeast infections, terrible PMS, depression, chronic fatigue syndrome, fibromyalgia, arthritis, and extreme exhaustion. And, as you're now aware, there's another symptom you can add to that list: weight gain.

Molds can grow anywhere there's moisture—indoors, outdoors, on wood, paper, carpets, food. But the most common toxic molds grow as black clumps on the walls, ceilings, or floors of buildings, including houses and apartments. Buildings can actually become "sick"—that is, infested—with mold.

Black mold is common in two parts of the country I'm very familiar with—Tennessee and Texas. But it's a serious issue everywhere. And the surprising thing is that it's more of a problem now than ever. It may be a result of modern buildings being more tightly sealed, allowing less ventilation. Also, air-conditioning systems may be unintentionally spreading mold spores to every nook and cranny of a structure.

Whatever the reason, I've found that approximately 50 percent of my sickest clients are living in mold-ridden homes or working in mold-ridden offices. I regularly treat entire families who have been exposed to toxic mold. One of the families had to have its home demolished. There was just no other way to stop the mold.

Another family was absolutely devastated by the effects of their mold-ridden house. The mother looked emaciated, the father was gaining weight at an alarming rate, and a daughter wasn't eating well or growing properly. It was horrible. We got them on nutrients, which helped considerably, but they had no choice but to move to another house. And guess what? The new house turned out to be just as mold-ridden. That should give you a pretty good idea of the magnitude of this problem.

Toxic Mold in the Schools

Tragically, the internal environment of many schools is "sick." My heart hurts when I think about how the health of so many of our young people has been compromised as a result. If your school-age children are often sick, consider the possibility that they're being sent to a toxic environment every day.

Just this past year, an elementary school in the Nashville area was closed down for mold infestation. This will become more and more of a problem and well known to the public over the next couple of years. In May 2002, State Farm Insurance issued an exception to all existing policies that they would no longer cover any damage from mold. It would be a good idea to check your home owner's insurance policy to see if you do in fact have coverage. The same concern applies to institutions of higher learning. I recently visited a college campus, where the dormitories were so badly mold-ridden that I could only take two steps into the hallway before needing to step back out. My work has made me keenly sensitive to toxic infestations, so I run out of moldy or contaminated buildings like I'm fleeing a fire. In this case, though, you didn't need to be an expert to know that the dorm wasn't healthy.

The good news, of course, is that you can avoid infested buildings and make sure your own home is mold-free. We'll get to that in Chapter Seven, but in the meantime, here's a tip: If it smells strong or offensive, it's toxic. Stay away from it. Again we have the God-given protective mechanism of being repulsed by certain smells. If you don't feel like being around a certain smell, the odds are there is a very good reason for that, and you need to remove yourself from it.

One of my clients is a college student, Mariah, who got back on her feet after we restored her to a health level she hadn't enjoyed for years. But soon after she went back to her classes, she was calling us in a toxic stupor. She eventually had to come home, unable to finish out the semester. We went back to the campus where she had been exposed, and sure enough, there was extensive mold in her living quarters. Not only that, her college was in a farming community where pesticides and fertilizer were constantly being sprayed. As I write this, Mariah is being taken through our intensive cleansing program. She has also chosen on her own not to return to that particular college. A wise decision, I must say.

HOME, TOXIC HOME

Mold is merely the most prominent of a smorgasbord of toxic substances in a typical home. I know this is not the most pleasant of topics, but it's essential that you become aware of the kinds of toxins you live with every day. So let's take a little tour around your home and pinpoint some typical toxic pitfalls.

The living room. Dust is the most common problem here, even that little bit you only worry about if your mother-in-law is coming to visit. For one thing, there's always more than you think. Just move a piece of furniture an inch or two, or take a couch pillow outside and beat it with a broom handle. You'll see what I mean.

Dust is full of mites and old dead skin cells that human bodies are sloughing off constantly. That means that in a dusty living room, you're breathing in your own toxins—and others'—over and over again.

Where there's lots of dust there's usually mold, since mold is great food for the dust mites. In fact, you may have already noticed that when a house smells dusty it's usually moldy, too. Which is a good example of how our sense of smell can warn us of toxic danger. One of your key assets in the Nashville Diet is your ability to listen to what your body is telling you. I'm going to ask you to work on that; it will help you adjust your nutrient doses, select healthy foods, and follow the detox plans (both internal and external) that I'll be outlining for you in the next two chapters. God gave us this ability, we just have to learn how to develop it by using the tools we already have.

One more living room hazard: The rugs or carpets themselves may be a problem, even if they're relatively dust-free. Studies have shown that fumes from new carpets are subtly toxic. On the other hand, if your carpet is old and musty-smelling, you may be dealing with mold.

The bedroom. You may be most vulnerable in the bedroom, where you probably spend at least a third of each day and where you tend to let your guard down. Dust is a big problem here too, but it's compounded by the fact that you sleep with your face and body pressed to sheets and blankets that may have collected any number of toxic substances from your body, your hair, your pet, your kids' clothes, and so on.

The kitchen. Now we're talking about a real toxic hot spot, especially if you keep cleaning chemicals and detergents under your sink. Solvents, such as the phenol in typical commercial cleaning formulas, are highly toxic, easily absorbed, and prone to take up long-term residence in your fat cells.

That old dishrag or sponge that you've used so often is by now solvent-soaked and likely to be dragging bacteria across your counters or dishes. Studies have actually shown that using kitchen rags is worse than eating off the kitchen floor!

Mold loves kitchens. Pipes that leak or let water seep out foster a fertile environment for mold growth. And refrigerators are infamous for their potential mold content.

The bathroom. Chances are you're storing (and using) more caustic cleaning solvents in your bathroom. Isn't there a faint but constant scent of synthetic cleaning agents in there? That's an indication that your system is receiving traces of chemicals that are toxic to it.

Bathrooms tend to stay wet, making them hospitable mold sites. And how about your toothbrush? You use it to remove bacteria from your mouth, and then leave it to spend the rest of its day as a breeding ground for more bacteria.

Now let's open up the vanity and explore the myriad modern toxins at home there. An antiperspirant's a must, right? Maybe so, but each time you apply it, you're infusing your systems with aluminum, a suspected culprit in Alzheimer's disease. You're also blocking the underarm's ability to serve as one of the main exit points of internal toxins.

Then there are the dozens of chemicals you spray on your hair to hold it in place. Perfume is another seemingly harmless toiletry that's full of toxins just waiting to be unleashed. The chemicals in the perfume smell nice, but they're poison to your body. There might also be harsh chemicals in your nail polish. Phthalates, chemicals found in many hairsprays, deodorants, and nail polishes, are suspected of causing birth defects. Whether they do or not, they surely add to your body's toxic burden.

Skin care products—with an endless variety of lotions, ointments, toners, and masques—also cause problems. When you rub chemical-laden products on your skin, it's like you're applying toxins directly into your body. Why? Because your skin is a giant, sophisticated "intake" system, as well as a means of excreting toxins. (Rarely does God provide us with anything for just one purpose!)

The skin's ability to "take in" substances from the outside is why pharmaceutical companies consider it one of the best drug-delivery methods. Creams, ointments, patches, and poultices are a few examples. So if something is just touching your skin—let alone being rubbed into it—it's going to end up in your bloodstream. So here's another rule of thumb for vibrant health: If you wouldn't eat it, don't put it on your skin.

The laundry room. This can be a virtual warehouse of toxic chemicals—in detergent, in fabric softeners, in bleach, in spray starch, and in most of the special cleaning agents you use from time to time. If you occasionally itch all over, consider your harsh crystallized detergent powder as a possible culprit.

The high toxicity of so many products commonly kept and used in bathrooms and laundry rooms is why so many maids and janitors come to my clinic. All of them are as sick and as fat as can be, but they get healthier and slimmer after we identify the source of their toxic overload, put them on the nutrients, and get them on a detoxification regimen. One woman (not a professional cleaner, but a housewife with lupus), responded beautifully to nutraplenishing and detox after she stopped cleaning her shower with bleach. She was able to get off her lupus medications and recover the healthy, trim body she hadn't had for twenty years.

The garage. Car exhaust, motor oil, brake fluid, gasoline . . . the list of common toxins in typical garages goes on and on. If you keep gardening supplies in there and you're in the habit of using chemical bug-killers and fertilizers, your garage (not to mention your garden) is that much more toxic. The garage is also another favorite site for mold growth. Some houses even have air-conditioning units in the garage that can circulate all those dangerous fumes throughout the house.

And you know that new-car smell we all like so much? That comes from carbon-based chemicals known as volatile organic compounds (VOCs), which easily vaporize and disperse into the air. One common VOC is benzene, often used in dyes and insecticides. It's a known carcinogen.

TOXINS IN YOUR FOOD

So far we've looked at three sources of toxins that contribute to your weight problems. One source consists of the toxic substances that are constantly generated as by-products of your body's internal processes. Your natural detoxification systems would be able to eliminate these toxins before they did much harm if (1) the systems were operating at full capacity, and (2) they didn't have to deal with so many additional toxins introduced from the outside.

The second source of toxins in your body is our polluted outdoor environment. That we're being persistently poisoned by smog, lead, industrial waste, dumped toxins, and contaminated waterways is so well known that I don't see the need to dwell much on it. Describing our toxic world is depressing enough without belaboring the obvious!

The third source is our indoor living and working spaces. As you've just learned, we cohabitate with toxins. The fact that so many of our indoor toxic enemies come from familiar items that we don't want to do without—such as perfume or laundry detergent—doesn't matter a wit to your crowded fat cells. As far as your body's concerned, toxins are toxins, and they must be dealt with if we're to get healthy and lean.

We will indeed be dealing with them very soon when we deploy our detox strategies. But first you need to be informed about a fourth source of toxic overload: the food you eat. Much as I hate to be the bearer of bad news (again!), our food is short on nutrients but often chock-full of toxins.

MEAT: THE PRICE OF PROTEIN

When we explored the nutrient-depleted state of our food supply back in the first chapter, you may have wondered why I didn't say anything about meat and other animal-based foods. The fact is that lean meat and dairy products do deliver certain nutrients we need and can't otherwise get in sufficient amounts. I respect vegetarianism, but I don't recommend it as part of the Nashville Diet.

Still, we need to be careful about the meat we eat because of its toxicity. For one thing, the chemicals that saturate our soils find their way into the fatty tissues of the animals we eat and end up in our own fatty tissue. Furthermore, most red meat is tinted with red dye—the very same stuff that makes kids hyperactive. It may also be bleached to extend its shelf life a little longer.

Far more dangerous, though, are all the toxic hormones and antibiotics shot into cattle and poultry to make them big and fat and commercially viable. You should know that most ranch animals don't lead anything close to natural lives. From their earliest days, they are altered by hormones and antibiotics, and grow up as much man-made toxic creations as God-made creatures. I'm no stranger to ranches, but it wasn't until a dear friend of mine told me about some strange cattle deaths that I realized just how extreme the hormone problem can be.

My friend drove a tractor-trailer and would often pull cattle to auctions. She was always aware that there was an urgent time factor in play as she rushed to get the cattle to the feed lots quickly so they could be sold and slaughtered. She assumed the time pressure had to do with saving money, with reducing the amount the cattle had to be fed and watered, and with limiting the time they spent standing around in their own feces.

But on one trip she was delayed by engine trouble and as time went on, the cattle started dropping dead! She was amazed. The weather wasn't hot, and there were no unusual conditions that might have been harming the herd.

When she solved the mystery, it was sobering news. It seems that in order to get the cattle to their maximum weight (and value), they would be pumped full of so many hormones just before shipment that it was just a matter of time before their livers would have to shut down. The idea was to time a lethal hormone dose for maximum effect just before the cattle were to be slaughtered anyway.

These hormones, which permeate all but the most carefully raised hormone-free cattle and swine are toxic to humans in any amount, and contribute to obesity. Think about it. Hormones cause cattle to literally blow up like balloons, which make them more valuable because beef is sold by the pound. Now doesn't it stand to reason that they are largely responsible for the weight gain in the Americans who are ingesting them with the meat they eat?

I also wonder just how much hormone-laden meat has to do with the fact that many young girls today are starting their periods at nine, eight, or even seven years old. I wonder: Is it connected with the fact that some boys are developing breasts? With the horrible problem of childhood obesity? With hormonal imbalances in women? With early menopause in women in their forties or even their thirties?

These are all serious problems that were not even issues forty years ago. New research investigating the causes, and possible connections with hormone-treated beef cattle, is extremely important. What I have found is that the timing of the start of America's health and obesity problems coincides very closely with the introduction of the pesticides, fertilizers, and especially the hormones in the meat and our love affair with fast food.

FISH: MERCURY RISING

Fish and shellfish are wonderful foods for most people. But they also contribute to our toxic overload. Fish swim in contaminated waters. So unfortunately for us, mercury (a toxin) is as common in fish as little bones are. The FDA, in fact, recommends that we limit our consumption of swordfish, shark, King mackerel, and Golden snapper (also known as tilefish) because of their mercury content.

The biggest problem, though, is with tuna, which is widely consumed in this country. Women are now being told to not eat more than one can of tuna per month while pregnant and breast-feeding. And if a pregnant woman is told to not do something, I would think that would be a good rule of thumb for the rest of us poor mortals. Also, remember that unclean or improperly cooked fish can deliver harmful bacteria.

PRODUCE: TOXINS—YES, NUTRIENTS—NO

I'm sure it will come as no surprise to you that chemical sprays and fertilizers do as much to raise your toxicity levels as they do to reduce the nutrient value of the food supply. Most people know that the fruits and vegetables we eat have been treated with synthetic chemicals. But I wonder how many are aware of just how much poison our food is subjected to.

There are hundreds of different pesticides and herbicides, and millions of tons of them are poured over fields and orchards every year.

The apple we came to know back in Chapter One is probably sprayed with toxic chemicals three or four times while it's on the tree. The nitrous oxide gas it's treated with upon picking is toxic, as is the dye that's applied to disguise the fact that it was harvested too early. It's sprayed again immediately after picking, and then again in the eighteen-wheeler that takes it to the wholesale market, where it's sprayed again. It will also get the bug-killer treatment at the retail store. By the time you eat it, that apple is loaded!

Processing in More Toxins

Any "fresh" fruit, vegetable, or whole grain you eat has been laced with enough toxins to keep your body's detox systems working overtime. But for much of the plant-based food we eat, those particular toxins are only half the story. That's because we get so much of our food in processed and packaged form, meaning it's been treated with any number of bleaching agents, emulsifiers, texturizers, humectants, and preservatives. There are literally thousands of different synthetic chemical food additives in use today. Most of them are made from petroleum or coal tar. All of them are toxic to our bodies.

Toxic Containers

As if we didn't have enough toxicity problems with our food, the actual packages they come in are often tainted. For example, the Centers for Disease Control in Atlanta once investigated soda cans and found that the tops were sometimes encrusted with dried rat urine. Pleasant thought, isn't it?

Almost everything you buy in a supermarket was stored in a warehouse at one time or another, and warehouses are often infested with rodents.

This is the reason that government regulations require that all these warehouses be continually sprayed with pesticides and the reason that "organic" can be "clean and pure" only so far. The food industry will have some difficult choices to make in the next few years. So if they're not properly cleaned before being put out on the aisles, the packaging of any foodstuffs can easily be contaminated with the residue of rat or mouse droppings, as well as toxic dust.

GENETICALLY ENGINEERED TOXINS

The aspect of the controversy about genetically engineered foods that most applies to our detox goals has to do with introduced chemicals. The most famous (and shocking) example was the corn that was genetically altered so that a pesticide would actually grow within the plant, rather than having to be sprayed on the crops. The FDA approved this poison corn only for cattle feed (as though that would make it harmless), but of course it ended up in the taco shells of a fast-food chain. Thank goodness somebody blew the whistle.

It may not seem like it, but I've really only given you a brief and partial list of the many toxins that find their way into our bodies. Trust me, I know how disturbing it can be to realize just how toxic our world is. But the lesson I want you to learn from all this is not one of doom and gloom. It's a lesson of hope. And it's the beginning of a plan of action. You *can* and *will* get those toxins under control, regain your vibrant health, and shed that excess fat—permanently.

Remember, it's my philosophy that vibrant health and a trim body are not achieved by blindly following the "instructions" of some fitness guru. Instead, they'll come from understanding your body and its needs, and learning how to take care of this wonderful gift from God.

If a fat-to-lean program is going to be of any value, you need to know what you're trying to do and why you're doing it. Toward that end, I believe that information is power. And I also believe that understanding any problem is the first step toward overcoming it.

You now have a basic understanding of the problem of toxicity and how it sabotages your weight-loss goals. Now let's get down to how to overcome it.

THE SOLUTION:

detoxification

as a child, I loved to visit my relatives' farm. My most enduring memory of those magical times has to do with the rain. Rain was a very big deal at that old farm. If it was heavy, it would flood the bottom land where the orchard trees grew, depositing nutrient-rich silt from the watershed to act as a natural fertilizer.

But what was good for the fruit trees wasn't so good for the bridge over the nearby stream at what we called the "low water crossing." Often the reservoir would rise too high behind the dam upstream, forcing the authorities to send water downstream. Whenever that happened, we'd be warned to prepare the low water crossing for a higher flow. That meant stripping out sediment and debris from the bridge area so the extra water would run smoothly under the bridge, not over it.

Whenever the warning call came, that old farm would spring into action. Bells would ring from the house and horns would honk from the rusted-out old trucks. People would drop whatever they were doing and go to work cleaning up the stream. Usually they'd get the job done in time, but once in a while they didn't make it. The bridge would be washed out, and it would take engineers days to get the concrete structure repaired and back into place.

My Aunt Goldie was the local authority on that bridge. She knew exactly what needed to be done to keep it from washing out. She also knew when it was safe for cars or pedestrians to cross it, and when it needed to be off-limits to one and all. Many "greenhorns" (as she called folks from other parts) had to be rescued from the flooded bridge after failing to heed Aunt Goldie's roadblocks.

At age twelve, I was one of those greenhorns. I'd meandered down to the forbidden low water crossing and lingered there, even as the bells rang and the horns honked. Suddenly I felt a blast of wind and looked up to see a wall of water roaring toward me. I gathered my wits and scurried off that bridge just as the water rushed over it. Only my left ankle was soaked, so I got off very cheaply compared to what might have happened. From that scary episode, I learned the price of carelessness, and of not listening to Aunt Goldie.

TARGETING THE TOXINS

To this day, I always think about that low water crossing when I help clients understand how to detoxify themselves. Since we live in a poisoned world, the "flow" of toxins into your body too often resembles the torrent of water in that old stream during rainstorms. Because toxins have accumulated inside you, your cells are like the stream bed itself, so overstuffed with debris and fill that it can't accommodate that extra flow. And because your lymphatic, digestive, and other natural toxin-eliminating systems are overworked and undernourished, they're like the washed-out bridge, in dire need of repair before they can function usefully.

I'm here to be your Aunt Goldie. I've already described the toxic problem, in full, gory detail. I've explained how it contributes to your weight problems. But like the real Aunt Goldie, I prefer taking action to wallowing in woe.

So let's get rid of those toxins. Let's defeat them by doing several things at once. Let's repair the bridge by nourishing our cells properly.

Let's clear out the junk under the bridge by purging our fat cells of accumulated toxins. And let's keep the stream flow down to a manageable level by drastically reducing our exposure to toxins.

I know it seems like a challenging undertaking. But you *can* detoxify, just as so many of my clients have done. And when you do, you'll have crossed the biggest barrier between fat and lean and sick and healthy.

NUTRAPLENISHING:
YOUR NUMBER ONE DETOXIFIER

Always be suspicious of any diet or health program that focuses on just one way to achieve success. There is no single thing that will get you from fat to lean. There's no lone magic bullet that delivers vibrant health. And there's certainly no one-shot solution to toxic overload.

In this chapter you'll learn a variety of detox techniques that you can put into action individually or practice together in what I call a "detox regimen." Then we'll move on to some very simple—but very important— changes you can introduce into your daily routine that will keep you away from the worst toxic sources and protect you from those toxins that cannot be avoided in today's world.

In other words, after decades of absorbing more toxins than your body can eliminate, you'll have plenty of new tools to take in less and move out more. But guess what? The first (and best) tool is one you're already familiar with—nutraplenishing. If you've started following the supplementation strategy I outlined in Chapter Four, you've already begun to detoxify.

YOUR NUTRIENTS COME FIRST

Cell nourishment by nutraplenishing is a mandatory prerequisite to any further detoxification steps. I want you to be on the nutrients for at least a month, with some significant gains in your Vibrant Health Index, before starting in on the detox techniques I'm about to give you.

The reason for this requirement is that only nutraceuticals can provide your body with the resources it needs to fight the toxins. It's very important to bring your body's systems closer to balance before releasing too many toxins from your fat cells. You want to make sure those freed-up toxins move into the detoxification pathways instead of simply relocating to areas where they can do more harm. The improved cellular performance that nutraplenishing brings will help get those toxins where they belong—out of your body.

Think of nutraplenishing as bridge repair and levee fortification to ensure proper channeling of the future flow of debris-laden stream water.

The toxin-fighting benefits you get from your nutraceutical regimen is known as "passive detoxification" because its primary purpose is to fortify your capacity to eliminate toxins rather than to attack toxins directly in specific organs or systems. But don't let that word "passive" fool you. Your nutrients are powerful detoxifiers that not only repair and reinforce, but also begin the process of clearing out accumulated toxins. They do this in a number of ways:

Your nutrients crowd out toxins. When you start taking nutraceuticals, you're delivering to your cells nutrients that have been AWOL for years or decades (because of our nutrient-depleted food supply). There's only so much space inside a cell, so to make room, the newly introduced nutrients often effectively kick out the toxins that had moved in uninvited. This is still considered passive detox, since the toxin expulsion is merely a by-product of the main task of cell building, but it definitely gets the ball rolling.

Your nutrients fight parasites. It's not for nothing that an entire category of your nutrient line-up is labeled Immune Boosters. Without a strong immune system, your body has difficulty processing parasites, bacteria, fungi, and viruses out of your system. They're all considered toxins, and we're continually exposed to them in the food we eat, the water we drink, and even the hands of the people who serve us that food and water. Your nutrients—especially the Immune Boosters but also the Detox Delights and certain others—help restore your body's ability to handle these pests.

Your nutrients neutralize free radicals. Unchecked oxidation from free radicals has been linked to a frightening number of major health problems, including asthma, muscle and bone damage, cataracts, immune deficiency, cardiovascular disease, and cancer. As you've already learned, our constant exposure to environmental toxins increases the body's production of free radicals, as do poor dietary habits. The good news is that a flood of recent scientific research has shown that the antioxidant properties of certain phytochemicals limit the danger from these "natural" toxins. The Fregetables nutraceuticals deliver precisely those antioxidants.

Your nutrients help your liver do its detox duties. If your liver function isn't sound, you're not healthy. One of many reasons the liver is so important is its role as the body's primary detoxifier. *Anything* absorbed during digestion passes through the liver to be cleared of toxins before entering the bloodstream. Obviously, if the liver is compromised in any way (which it easily can be if overwhelmed by toxins, including alcohol), your overall toxicity will rise. That's why the liver tonic herbs you're taking—dandelion, turmeric, and milk thistle—are key detox nutrients.

Your nutrients replenish your cells. Delivering nutrients to your cells by nutraplenishing takes on added importance as you move to more active detox techniques. As you flush out more toxins, some non-toxic and vital cell matter will inevitably go out with them. Your nutrients compensate for that loss, replenishing the good stuff that gets flushed out with the bad stuff.

PRIMARY TARGET: THE COLON

There are yet more toxin fighters in your nutrients. I consider their particular detox effects to be closer to the "active" end of the action scale because they're aimed at a specific target—the colon.

Active detoxification should start with colon cleansing. As I'm sure you're aware, it's through the colon that waste matter and the toxins it carries exit the premises. But your gastrointestinal tract in general and your colon in particular are among the likeliest places for your body to break down, creating blockage that impedes elimination. Shocking as it may sound; it's not uncommon for an adult bowel to retain ten or more pounds of old toxin-laden fecal matter.

Bowel movements are by no means the only way your body rids itself of toxins. Toxins can be eliminated through skin, breath, and urine. They can be neutralized or transformed by internal chemical reactions. But a poorly functioning gastrointestinal tract, which houses a majority of your immune system, will "retoxify" the rest of your body, canceling out any other detoxification efforts you may be making.

Also, when your food is not properly broken down, absorbed, utilized, and eliminated, you build more unhealthy fat and cellulite. You're more tired after you eat, instead of feeling energized. Additionally, most Americans harbor intestinal parasites, which can cause a host of seemingly unrelated problems and general discomfort.

For all these reasons, it's critical to first work on detoxifying your entire digestive tract, starting with your colon. The nutrients in the Detox Delights category do exactly that. Here's how:

Detox Delights fight pests. Some of these nutrients in effect make your digestive system taste bad to mold, candida, parasites, microbes, and similar organisms by changing the acid–base balance in your gastrointestinal tract. The pests simply stop "eating," and over a period of time die and are eliminated by your system. Your immune system builds up as a result, and you find that your strength gradually increases and food cravings gradually disappear.

Detox Delights encourage bowel movements. You must have at least one bowel movement per day to maintain a healthy weight. The entire digestive process begins as soon as you start chewing, and ends (ideally) thirty minutes later with a bowel movement. My guess is that this is not happening with you on schedule, but by taking the Detox Delights according to the program I've given you, and drinking plenty of water, you'll soon develop much healthier elimination schedules.

These nutrients deliver insoluble fiber that is absorbed directly into your gastrointestinal system, providing the bulk you need to keep things moving along.

Detox Delights eliminate accumulated waste. Because the fiber in these nutrients stimulates the muscle in your bowels and intestines, it helps break loose all the old decaying toxins that have built up over the years, and replaces them with immune-replenishing nourishment. You'll notice the resulting strength, energy, and clean, fresh feeling you get as a result of just this component of your nutrient regimen.

Detox Delights improve overall digestion. The digestion issue was an important area for me to address personally. When I first began my nutrients, I had to take unbelievable amounts of the best products I could find to even begin to digest my foods. Either I would not eliminate for weeks or I would force my digestive system so much that my system would eliminate whole food without breaking it down. I was so out of whack that there was some concern that I had gastrointestinal cancer or something equally serious. My digestion finally improved when I found the best combination of nutrients for the digestive system—which I have now passed along to you.

With so many toxins in the food and environment, the chances are good that you're continually exposing your gastrointestinal system to carcinogens and parasites. This creates a cascade effect in which more and more toxins are deposited in your system, which becomes less and less able to handle them. The combination of nutrients in your Detox Delights turns things around by killing harmful parasites, replenishing good bacteria, dislodging accumulated fecal waste, stimulating the bowel and intestinal muscles, and helping toxin elimination by nourishing the cells of your entire digestive tract.

By restoring the health of your colon and the rest of your digestive tract, the Detox Delights allow your body to break down food properly so that it can be used to build up health instead of break it down. And even as they do all that, these nutrients deliver another wonderful benefit for your fat-to-lean quest. You'll find that as you take these capsules, your appetite will decrease. Which makes sense, doesn't it? When food is processed efficiently, your body demands less of it.

LOVE YOUR NUTRIENTS!

The lesson so far is that nutraplenishing is not only the key to restoring your cell function and eliminating food cravings, but also the foundation for ridding your body of accumulated toxins. For a lucky few who are extremely healthy even as they're somewhat overweight, nutraplenishing might be all the detox they need. For the rest (the vast majority), the detox strategies I'm about to describe will work wonders.

But everybody needs to be diligent about taking their nutrients every day. You need to keep taking them even though you're not losing a significant amount of weight in the early stages. Remember, the Nashville Diet is not a quickie weight-loss scheme that moves the scale needle down the first week to give you a false sense of achieving something permanent. Instead, you're giving your body the ability to easily get to its best weight and stay there. You're doing this by restoring your cellular function after years of nutrient deprivation, and shrinking your fat cells by ridding them of accumulated toxins.

Both these stages depend on nutraplenishing. I cannot urge you enough to keep taking your nutrients, and to stay faithful to the supplementation plan you learned in Chapter Four. Those nutrients are the best friends your body has had in a long time.

Easy Does It

Before I give you some active detoxification techniques, I'm going to establish two detoxification rules: (1) Go slow, and (2) take things one step at a time.

Both of my rules require patience. Detoxifying your body isn't like brushing crumbs off a table. After all, you're dealing with poisons. Your toxicity level has been built cell by cell, layer upon layer, for years. You must reduce it the same way. Push too hard and you'll find yourself in extreme discomfort.

Remember, you're actually following two simultaneous paths to detoxify. You're rebuilding healthy cells via nutraplenishing. You're also chipping away at the toxic overload by the more active detox actions of some of the nutrients, as well as the techniques that follow. Allow your body time for the internal cell building and the exterior toxic burn to meet in the middle.

The changes will be steady but subtle during your detox phase. You probably won't see the scales move much, since you're concentrating on eliminating toxins. But look out! When your system does get cleaned out and your cells have progressed in their building of new and healthy tissue—that's when your metabolism kicks into overdrive, and the fat will start to melt away. When that happens, you will no longer look, feel, or act like the same person.

One Step at a Time

Unlike fad diets, the Nashville Diet moves ahead in bite-size chunks, taking one thing at a time. You've already seen this philosophy in action in the way you built up in stages to your permanent nutraplenishing plan. It's also reflected in my requirement that you nutraplenish for at least a month before moving on to the more aggressive detox program in this chapter and the next.

One reason for this incremental approach is to make things more practical for you. I understand how all this new information about your undernourished cells and toxic overload can seem overwhelming. Believe me, I went through it. Then to actually embark on a new nutraplenishing and detox programs to overcome those problems...well, it's a tall order, even though you know it's the best way to get permanently healthy and lean. Sticking with small, easy steps is the best way to deal with the challenge.

But there's an even more important reason to pace yourself as you detox. The toxins must be released from their hiding places at a manageable rate. The last thing you want to do is liberate a flood of toxins into your bloodstream all at once. If you're going to stir up toxins, they'd better have a way out of your body. Your lymphatic system, your liver, and other toxin-elimination pathways must be able to handle the increased load. If not, the toxins will simply find a new home and you'll feel the unpleasant effects.

This "autointoxication," brought on by letting loose too many toxins in too short a time, is communicated to you in the language of pain. You might suffer headaches, abdominal cramps, flu-like symptoms, or a skin rash. Going slow is generally your best defense against autointoxication, but different people respond differently to active detox. Listen to your body. If something abnormal arises, take a step back. Hold off on your last detox technique. You may even have moved too far ahead on your nutrient dosage. Remember, you're never wasting time by making a tactical retreat. You're simply respecting your body's pace while learning to listen to what your body is trying to tell you.

Your VHI Is Your Detox Guide

To repeat, you should be nutraplenishing for at least a month before undertaking the detox regimen below. I say "at least" because some people are still not internally strong enough for active detox even after a month of nutraplenishing. How do you know? By consulting your latest VHI score.

☐ If your VHI is below 50, you're not ready for active detox. Your detoxification pathways—kidney, liver, lymphatic system, skin, and so on—won't be able to usher out the freed-up toxins. Continue with your passive detox by staying on the nutraplenishing regimen that's appropriate for you.

- ☐ If your VHI is between 50 and 60, you must limit yourself
   to just a few of the techniques below. You'll learn which
   ones you can do as they're described.
- ☐ If your VHI is between 60 and 75, approach your active
   detox with much caution. Go extra slow. If you experience
   any discomfort or difficulty, retreat to just nutraplenishing
   and come back stronger in a week or two.
- ☐ If your VHI is 75 or more, congratulations! You're definitely ready to get those toxins out of the way so you can
   get lean and healthy. Take it easy, though. You may have
   a head start, but this isn't a fifty-yard dash. It's more like a
   marathon, in that you'll need to use your resources slowly
   and consistently.

DETOX TECHNIQUES

I've placed so much emphasis on the importance of detoxifying your systems that it may surprise you how simple most of the following techniques
are. Nevertheless, when practiced in conjunction with your nutraplenishing, these activities will help your body steadily rid itself of accumulated toxins and become ready to let go of fat.

These techniques focus on your lymphatic system, which you can
think of as your body's toxic waste disposal service. The lymphatic system
consists of "tubes" that course like veins through your body. Running
through the tubes is a fluid that carries toxins away. Unlike your bloodstream, the lymphatic fluid isn't pumped through the tubes but rather is
induced to move through a system of one-way valves by muscle contractions and your body's movements. Your goal is to get the lymphatic fluid
moving to flush those toxins out of your body. The techniques also help
by flushing excess toxins out of the lymphatic system and into the bloodstream for processing through other detox pathways, thereby breaking log-
jams in the lymphatic system.

Lymphatic Massage

Why it works.

Massaging action slowly dislodges toxins trapped in the lymphatic system, which are eventually released into the bloodstream and processed by the kidney, liver, and bowels.

What to do.

Bring the fingers of both hands to a spot on the left and right sides of your neck, just above the clavicle (collar bone) and below the larynx (Adam's apple). Massage *gently* in tiny inward circles for one minute. Make sure you don't massage too hard, or the lymphatic system will simply shut down.

When to do it.

Perform the lymphatic massage for one minute before getting out of bed in the morning, while you're still groggy. Do it again for thirty seconds at night just before sleep.

VHI requirement.

Good for all VHIs over 50. Sometimes you might feel a bit light-headed after the massage. That's merely an indication that your lymphatic system is being cleared.

Diaphragmatic Breathing

Why it works.

Enriching the oxygen supply throughout the body opens your toxin-clearing pathways.

What to do.

Take in a long, slow, deep breath through your nose, letting it fill your belly first and then work its way upward. It should look like a baby's breath, with the tummy actually moving out as you breathe in. Keep drawing your breath in until you can no longer fill your lungs. Then push out hard through your mouth.

When to do it.
Take two prolonged diaphragmatic breaths after your lymphatic massage in bed in the morning.

VHI requirement.
Good for all VHIs.

LEMON PUSH

Why it works.
Lemon acts as an expectorant, breaking down and liquefying mucus to more easily push it and the toxins it contains out of the system. As a diuretic, lemon also pulls toxins from the kidneys to release them in the urine.

What to do.
The idea is to deliver a lot of lemon quickly to maximize detoxification. Squeeze a whole fresh lemon into 16 ounces of distilled water and drink it down all at once. Then drink another glass of distilled water immediately after drinking the lemon water. This is the "push." This much water will break loose any toxins and wash them out of your system.

When to do it.
Do one lemon push in the morning before breakfast.

VHI requirement.
Good for VHIs 60 and over. The most important requirement is that you faithfully take your nutrients. Lemon pushes are like strip-mining, because the lemon attaches to good minerals and nutrients as well as the toxins. You need to make sure those lost nutrients are replaced.

DRY SKIN BRUSH

Why it works.

Right alongside the millions of tiny blood vessels or capillaries just beneath the surface of your skin run similarly tiny lymphatic system tubes. Stimulating the skin by brushing moves excess toxins out of these extremities of your lymphatic system and into the bloodstream for processing and elimination.

Furthermore, because your skin is an exit point for certain toxins, shedding dead skin cells is important for detoxification. Dry skin brushing helps get rid of unseen excess dead skin layers, and the toxins they contain.

What to do.

Buy two natural-bristle skin brushes, one slightly softer for facial use. Using short movements, brush your entire body for five to ten minutes, depending on your VHI. For all skin above the waist, brush toward the base of your neck. That means the brush strokes on your face will be downward, while all other strokes from the waist up will go upward. Brush your arms from your fingertips toward your shoulders. From the waist down, brush toward your groin area, meaning all the strokes except those on the highest part of your waist will be upward.

When to do it.

Any time of day is fine, but make sure your skin is completely dry when you brush it. Brushing wet skin causes it to stretch, encouraging wrinkles. That means brushing during a shower is out. In case you're wondering, using a loofah sponge while bathing does not have the same detoxifying effect.

VHI requirement.

If your VHI is over 70, brush for ten minutes. If your VHI is 60 to 70, brush for seven minutes. If your VHI is 50 to 60, brush for five minutes. Do not do the dry skin brush if your VHI is below 50.

TAI CHI

Why it works.

This gentle and accessible Chinese martial art promotes inner strength and purity by integrating breathing, physical movement, mental concentration, and visual awareness. The circular, relaxed, fluid movements stimulate blood circulation and the movement of the lymphatic fluids.

What to do.

There are people, of course, who dedicate a large chunk of their lives to mastering tai chi. I do recommend that you take advantage of the widespread availability of tai chi classes in health clubs, community centers, and martial arts studios in just about every town across the country. There are also many good books on the subject, as well as videos. For the purpose of your detoxifying efforts, however, I've adapted a simplified four-stage "home version" that will bring excellent results.

Stage 1—Breathe. The foundation of tai chi is breathing. The tai chi breathing technique you'll use is much the same as the diaphragmatic breathing exercises you do in the morning. Breathe in deeply, filling first the belly and then the lungs to capacity. Your exhale won't be as sudden as in diaphragmatic breathing. Watch yourself in a mirror to make sure your chest and abdomen expand, but your shoulders stay stable. You'll use this breathing style when you perform simple tai chi movements, inhaling to prepare for the motion, exhaling when making the movement, and inhaling again between movements.

Stage 2—Relax. First, relax every muscle in your body. Now tighten just your right biceps (the muscle on the front of your upper arm when your palm is face up). Look at your hand. Is your fist clenched? Try again and think about every muscle being relaxed except for your right biceps.

Stage 3—Align. Practice alignment in front of a mirror. The goal is to stabilize your torso from your waist to your shoulders. You'll need to focus on the entire inner lower torso, specifically the stomach-area muscles (the abdominals), and the lower back muscles that support your spine (the erector spinae). Lift your shoulders and roll them back so your shoulder blades are pulled together behind you. Position your chin parallel to the floor. Tilt your chest outward. Tuck your hips under your naturally contracted abdominals. Your feet are shoulder-width apart and your knees are just slightly bent. Now you're aligned. But are you comfortable? Of course not! You probably haven't been in anything like this position since high school gym class. Your task at this stage is to simply take a few minutes every day to get comfortable in this position.

Stage 4—Energize. Now you're ready to perform some easy tai chi movements that have a detoxifying effect (among many other benefits). No matter which part of your body you're moving, tai chi movements pair actions with their apparent opposites. The Chinese apply the same terms for these pairs (yin and yang) that they do for other opposites in life—light and dark, up and down, hot and cold. The yin movements are softer, work with gravity, and are considered "empty." The yang movements are harder, work against gravity, and are often called "full." A goal of tai chi is to let the yin and yang movements flow together even as you're constantly shifting between the two.

Tai chi movements. To start a movement, you need to get rooted to facilitate the circular nature of the motions. This is where your Stage 3 alignment practice pays off, although you'll want to bend your knees slightly more. Then visualize the movement before you start it. There's nothing mystical about this visualization. Simply picturing the movement before you do it helps your mind and body work better together, and lets you perform the movement more confidently.

Here are some movements to try. Practice the arm and leg movements separately until you can do them smoothly and fluidly. Then try to combine them.

Arms. Hold your arms out in front of you with your palms facing each other, letting your fingers and elbows soften as you imagine holding a large ball between your hands. (1) Keep holding the ball as you slowly raise your arms up while breathing in. Breathe out as you slowly lower the ball again. (2) Slowly bring the imaginary ball to your chest by moving your elbows behind you as you breathe in, and then breathe out as you push the ball back out. (3) Now imagine that you're holding medium-size balls in each hand, and slowly open your arms wide while breathing in, then bring them back together while breathing out.

Legs—Bow stance. From your aligned posture position, turn your right toe out slightly and bend your right knee a little so that it bears all your weight. Raise your left knee and step out to the front, landing with your left heel and then rolling the rest of your foot down flat. Your position now looks like a lunge. Reverse the motion to return to the original position, and repeat on the other side. Remember to breathe in during the positive motion and out as you return. Work on making the entire movement fluid and continuous, rather than jerky.

Legs—Empty step. From your aligned posture position, breathe out as you take one step directly forward with your left foot. Shift your weight to your back leg and bend both knees as far as you can. Breathe out as you return and repeat with the other foot.

The first thing you'll probably notice as you try the movements is that they're harder than they sound. Don't be surprised if you're wobbly. No problem! If you feel off balance, just stop and try again. It may take weeks or months to master these movements. It doesn't matter. The effort alone is beneficial.

When to do it.

Practice for five to ten minutes a day, but don't try to do everything at once. For your first sessions, you may practice only breathing and relaxation. Then you may work on your alignment. Perhaps you'll have several sessions under your belt before you begin to tackle the movements. Remember, it's not a race. Each time you practice, you're chiseling away at your toxicity level.

REBOUND JUMPING

Why it works.

The up-and-down activity of this "miniature trampoline" exercise stimulates the opening and closing of the one-way valves of the lymphatic system, significantly increasing your lymph flow. This creates a suction effect at the millions of lymphatic terminals throughout your body, moving toxins out of your fat cells and into your waste disposal system. Because of the toxin-clearing effects of the other techniques you're practicing, your lymphatic system is better able to handle the additional toxins.

What to do.

Buy yourself a mini-trampoline at any sporting goods store, specifying that you need one appropriate for rebounding exercise. They're not very expensive and well worth the investment. Then start practicing the following bouncing techniques, presented here in ascending order of difficulty.

The health bounce. This is shallow, up-and-down bouncing; your toes never leave the surface of the trampoline.

The aerobic bounce. Here you're walking, jogging, or even semi-sprinting in place. But again, no jumping. Let there be no air between your toes and the trampoline surface.

The strength bounce. Jump straight up and down, letting your feet come off the surface each time. Don't try to jump too high—just enough to get some air between your feet and the trampoline surface.

When to do it.
Practice rebounding five days a week for two to twenty minutes, depending on your VHI and your conditioning level. Allow at least ten minutes of rest before eating after a bouncing session.

VHI requirements.
Rebounding is a highly detoxifying exercise that's not recommended for those with VHIs under 60. If your VHI is 60 to 65, start off with just two minutes of the health bounce only. If your VHI is between 65 and 70, do two minutes of each of the bounces, for a total of six minutes.

HYDROTHERAPY

Why it works.
Hydrotherapy is a scientific-sounding name that for our purposes is a fairly simple hot-and-cold–water treatment you do in the shower to improve your circulation. The hot water dilates the blood vessels so they can better accept the toxic overflow from the loosened lymphatic system. The cold water clamps the blood vessels down, constricting them and forcing the toxins to move through to where they can be processed for elimination.

What to do.
Don't expect a relaxing shower. Start with three minutes of very hot water. Increase the temperature until it's as hot as you can stand it and then increase it a little more. Don't cheat yourself! Follow that up with one minute of cold water, as cold as you can get it.

Eventually you want to repeat this four-minute cycle seven times, but you'll have to work your way up to that. You may also have to work your way up to the maximum hot and cold temperatures. If you are doing it correctly, you'll get a taste of salt in your mouth during the third or fourth cycle. Also, when you get up to four cycles, you may find that you can't tell the difference between the hot and cold water after the third cycle. Then you know it's working.

When to do it.

This is an intensive detoxifier that need not be done daily, except for the three-week period in which you follow the complete detox regimen. Logically, you'd do it during your daily shower. One problem is that you can run through your hot water supply before the full twenty-eight minutes are up. If so, don't worry about it. There's plenty of detox benefit in just one or two cycles.

VHI requirements.

This hydrotherapy technique is not for those with VHIs under 50. If your VHI is under 70, you'll need to work your way up very slowly to maximum temperature and duration.

PUTTING IT ALL TOGETHER

I've just given you seven detox techniques to practice, and it probably feels like a thousand. I'm willing to bet you never expected to be involved with tai chi, a trampoline, and hydrotherapy all at the same time! But these are all very effective detoxifying exercises that my clients rave about once they get used to them. And of course they love the way fat starts to melt away once they've brought their toxicity down to healthy levels.

The secret to success is in the two rules I gave you at the outset—go slow and take things a step at a time. Start off with one of the techniques. As you begin to make progress with it, incorporate another technique. Add techniques one at a time, but drop the latest one if you experience unpleasant symptoms. Once you feel better, try to edge forward again.

When you're comfortable with (although not necessarily an expert at) all seven techniques, you're ready for a one-time-only, three-week routine incorporating the entire regimen. This is like an overhaul of your systems, an intense detox course that will catapult you ahead to the next phase of the Nashville Diet. It consists of performing all seven of the detox techniques once a day for three weeks.

This is a tall order, but definitely doable. Your VHI should be over 70. You should be able to perform the techniques without discomfort. And you should be motivated and eager to follow the routine. If you dread the idea of doing it, you're better off working through selected cleansing techniques at your own pace.

Once you've put yourself through the three-week cleansing regimen, it's time to ease up on the detox techniques. Of course, you'll continue to take your nutrients. You may want to continue practicing tai chi for all its mental and physical health benefits. Rebounding may continue to be your chosen form of aerobic exercise, which we'll be getting into in the next chapter. Also, the early-morning diaphragmatic breathing is something you can do for the rest of your life. But the lemon pushes, dry skin brushes, lymphatic massages, and hydrotherapy should be relegated to an occasional, as-needed basis. After one to three months of detox exercises and nutraplenishing, along with the lifestyle tricks you'll learn in the next chapter, you'll feel healthier and more energetic. You'll also notice that some fat has disappeared. Most importantly, your toxicity will have decreased to a point where you're ready to start losing some serious weight!

the detox lifestyle

feeling better? I wouldn't be surprised if you do, even if all you've done so far is read. Here's why:

You're now familiar with two pillars of the Nashville Diet that virtually no other weight-loss strategy even considers, let alone focuses on. One is the absolute necessity of limiting your food cravings by nourishing your cells far beyond what our food supply is capable of. The other is the importance of drastically reducing your internal toxicity to clear the way for your body to let go of fat.

What makes this a truly breakthrough approach to fat loss is that the central strategy of the Nashville Diet—nutraplenishing—achieves both those goals. A daily regimen of nutraceuticals in the form of capsulated concentrated food gets your cells the vital nutrients they've been demanding for so long. And it begins the process of easing toxins out of your fat cells and restoring your systems' ability to flush those fat-favoring toxins out of your body.

So far, we've looked at two weapons for you to use against toxicity. Besides nutraplenishing, you'll be helping your body rid itself of long-stored toxins by introducing into your life the simple detox techniques I described for you in the last chapter. In Part Three, you'll learn how smarter food choices will complete your detox assignment as you accelerate down the lean-bound highway.

In the meantime, though, you and I are still living in a poisoned world. Even as we take steps to rid our bodies of accumulated toxins, we're soaking in more every day. Can we do anything to reduce our toxic exposure and stay ahead of the detox game? You bet we can.

We've talked about all the toxins within you and without you. In this chapter I'll show you how to fortify yourself against some of the most common toxins you're faced with—by purifying your home environment, cleansing your system with pure, clean water, and weaning yourself safely and carefully from prescription medications.

TOXIC HOUSE GUESTS

Maybe our great-grandchildren will live in a world where they won't be taking in toxins just by stepping outside. We don't. But we can greatly reduce toxin accumulations in our bodies by making some adjustments indoors.

MOLD IS YOUR FIRST ORDER OF BUSINESS

I can't tell you how many clients of mine made stunning progress after they had their homes checked for mold—and then cleaned it up. The story is often the same: A desperate client seeks my help. She begins to feel better, and drops some dress sizes as her nutraplenishing program progresses. But then she hits a wall and just can't seem to lose the remaining excess weight and recover her full vibrant health. That's when we start looking for ongoing sources of toxic exposure, and we usually find it in the form of a mold-ridden home. The top priority immediately becomes getting that mold away from the client (or getting the client away from the mold). The positive results are amazing.

Experts pay a lot more attention to the dangers of household mold these days. But in my experience, average people think of mold as more of a nuisance than the health threat it really is. Most of my clients are stunned when I trace their weight and health troubles to mold in their homes. They never considered such a thing as a possible culprit. Does that sound like you? If so, I urge you to change your thinking and make mold eradication a top priority.

If your house or apartment building is more than four years old, consider that age a red flag for possible mold problems. If you're aware of a constant musty or dusty smell in your home, consider that a blaring warning siren. You need to investigate. Here's what you can do.

Check for leaks. Most home mold infestations start around a leak under the kitchen sink or from the dishwasher, just about anywhere in the bathroom, or from the roof.

Clean after you fix. Having someone come in and fix the leak is great, but not enough. Mold may have already started growing like a cancer, and it won't stop just because the leak is fixed. Go at it with full-strength bleach and brushes, making sure you dry it thoroughly. Be sure to wear a mask and have good ventilation.

Replace what you can't clean. You must get rid of all the mold, but that's not always possible by cleaning. Not all mold can be cleaned away. Anything that's absorbent—like floor tiles or ceiling tiles, bare wood, rugs, carpets, etc. —will probably have to be replaced.

Search the garage and basement. Don't make the mistake of considering these spaces as something apart from where you actually live. Any time spent there is enough to contaminate you, and spores from garage mold can easily make their way into the main part of your home through the ventilation system. Even the process of coming and going in and out of the house can allow the toxins in.

Prevent mold in the first place. Make it a point to keep potential problem areas dry as well as clean. Dry behind appliances, along baseboards, on and under carpets and furniture, and inside the refrigerator. Keep your bathroom well ventilated, with a fan if necessary, and dry up that bath water or sink water that always spills over no matter how careful you try to be. Use your kitchen exhaust fan not just while cooking but also while washing the dishes and cleaning.

Use an expert. The truth is, household mold is sometimes too complicated a problem for laypersons to handle. And it's so potentially devastating to your health that it's definitely better to be safe than sorry. So if you suspect your home might have a mold problem, take advantage of the growing number of "mold remediation" professionals who'll check your home for infestation and supervise the cleanup. I have one come into my home at least once a year as a matter of routine.

HOME, SAFE HOME: DETECTING RADON

You can't see radon. You can't smell it or feel it, either. What you *can* do is test for it. As with mold, you can call in an expert to determine whether radon is a problem in your house. When you're buying a new home, an expert evaluation is a must. For the home you're already in, you can order a do-it-yourself test kit from the National Safety Council at (800) 557-2366. You simply follow the instructions, and then send the kit to a laboratory for the results.

Here are some other home suggestions.

Change your air conditioner and furnace filters regularly. These filters usually come with a recommended life span. Be sure to replace them as often as the manufacturer recommends. And don't economize on these filters; go for the most efficient available. For air conditioning, I recommend air filters that have a sticky substance on them; they catch much more than the cheaper, throwaway kind. They'll last three to four months. But they do have to be vacuumed out once a month, minimum.

Have your air-conditioning system serviced at the beginning of each season. Before you turn on the air conditioning for the first time each year, make sure it's serviced and working properly. There is a "trap" in the unit that's intentionally filled with water to make sure that the smell and bacteria from the sewer doesn't back up into your home through the air-conditioning system. But sitting water always means mold, not to mention all kinds of bacteria and other organisms that can grow there. To solve the problem, you can drop a large bleach tablet into the water trap to stop mold from growing. This is a good idea especially if you have centralized air conditioning. Just remember that as you start the system back up when hot weather returns, bleach-contaminated air will blow out for a brief period. You can get around that by going away for a few days and having a heating and air-conditioning company come out to flush the lines and run the unit for a couple days while you're away.

Leave your home during toxin-stirring procedures. If you have your heating or air conditioning serviced, get out of the house, and stay out of there until the coast (or house) is clear. The same theory applies if you have your floors treated (sanded, varnished, etc.).

One of my most toxic clients had been housebound and bedridden for years before she got out of her toxic fog, thanks to nutrients, her internal environment cleanup, and having her house demolded. She shrank five sizes and got off her asthma medication. Then she decided to have her heating and air-conditioning systems serviced. The moment I heard about it, I called to make sure she'd get out of that house for at least three days. Too late. She'd stayed in the house for two days after the servicing. I knew what was coming next.

And sure enough, she told me shortly after, "I've been sick ever since they serviced my central system. I'm still mentally here, but I feel bad again." She developed histoplasmosis in her lungs. We were able to get her back on her feet again, but it took time and pain—which she wouldn't have had to go through had she taken the precautions I'm giving you here. Knowing about toxins isn't enough; you must heed the warnings.

Install a carbon monoxide detector on each floor of your home. These detectors can be installed just like a typical smoke alarm. You can buy them wherever you buy smoke alarms, such as at home improvement stores.

Protect yourself and your family from formaldehyde.
Stick with solid wood furniture instead of particle board or fiberboard.

Air out new carpeting before installation. Any new carpeting
should be aired for several days before being laid down in your home.
Then it needs to be cleaned by experts, even though it's brand new. I've
had lots of clients who do great after years of frustration with health and
weight issues, but then go down like a sliding piano as soon as they install
new carpets or move into a brand new home. There are so many toxins in
"new stuff" like carpeting, cabinets, and new Sheetrock with new paint
that it would be impossible to name them all here. The two worst are the
formaldehyde and the toluene in the dyes.

"Burn out" your new house. That spanking-new, just-built
house you're about to move into is full of debris like Sheetrock dust, much
of it in the vents. Here are some very effective steps you can take to eliminate poisonous toxins before you have that housewarming party.

Before you move into your new house, have the entire ventilation
system vacuumed out by professionals. Then leave it sealed up for three
days with the heat on as high as it will go. What this does is accelerate the
"off-gassing" process that would normally take three years, soaking you
with toxins all that time. As these new, manmade products are exposed to
oxygen, a chemical reaction occurs that causes them to expel some of the
poisonous gases and materials they were made with into the air that you're
living in and breathing, thus the term off-gassing. This term literally
means putting off gasses, and in this case they are poisonous gases. You
know this is happening because you can smell it—that new-house smell
or that new-car smell. This heating up simply accelerates this process. The
burn out literally boils off the toxic fumes in a short period of time. You
definitely do *not* want to enter the house in such a state. But once the
doors are all opened, then have an expert that is suited up enter and open
all the windows. Leave everything open for about an hour, then you can
enter your now toxin-free house.

Enforce a strict no-smoking rule in your house. Few guests
these days will be offended by this.

CLEANING WITHOUT TOXIFYING

You have a Catch-22 problem in your home. You need to keep it clean, but as we've seen, most common household cleaning products are chemical cauldrons that soak your cells with toxins. You can't completely avoid solvents and other harmful substances, but you can cut down your toxic exposure considerably by taking some simple precautions.

First of all, if you send laundry out, remember that dry cleaning really means cleaning with chemicals. Take those dry-cleaned clothes out of that plastic bag and let them hang in fresh air for two hours before you hang them up.

At home, protect yourself whenever you use any kind of cleanser. We go to great lengths to keep chemicals away from our children, but then we let those same chemicals seep into our own skin. Use strong rubber gloves, and make sure you have adequate ventilation.

Then consider substituting some of the following less-harmful cleansing solutions for the commercial cleansers you're used to. Bear in mind that many of them may not work as quickly or efficiently as conventional products. And it's possible that you can experience allergic reactions or other negative side effects from substances that are new to you. So don't run out and buy every one of the alternatives and overhaul your entire routine all at once. First try one, then another, and see how things go. Remember, any reduction in your toxic exposure is worthwhile.

Instead of disinfectant...
>   use half a cup of borax in one gallon of hot water.

Instead of powdered laundry detergent...
>   use borax or liquid detergents. Powdered detergents have phosphates in them that borax and liquid detergents do not have. My personal favorites are liquid Dreft or Ivory. Both of these have a little bit of scent in them and if you still have problems with allergies, you're better off to stick with borax. Rinse your sheets and pillowcases twice, using hot water, and dry them in high heat.

Instead of drain cleaners...

use a flushing mixture of equal parts baking soda and vinegar (about ¼ cup each) in some water. If you have a food processor or juicer you can juice or blend citric fruit peels, like grapefruit, oranges, or lemons. Put it in your clogged toilet or other drain and let it sit. Then wash it down with hot water. Bonus: It smells good.

Instead of bleach...

try lemon juice or borax. If only bleach will do, choose an oxygen-based bleach such as hydrogen peroxide. Hydrogen peroxide literally turns to water when it is mixed with water. In the few seconds it takes for this process to happen it can whiten your clothes. Chlorine bleach has chlorine, which starts out as a very concentrated halogen gas. This is used to kill many germs, so it can kill the "good bacteria" in your system, along with the living cells in your immune system.

Instead of ant spray...

clean away the ants and sprinkle chile powder in the area. Seal all possible ant entry points with caulk.

Instead of furniture polish...

wipe with almond oil or olive oil.

Instead of stainless steel cleaner...

use baking soda in a little bit of water.

Instead of toilet bowl cleaner...

scrub with baking soda and castile soap or use the "juice" from citrus fruit peels. You can leave it to clean for itself and have a great-smelling bathroom at the same time.

Instead of window cleaner...

mix half a cup of vinegar in a quart of warm water for inside windows. For outside windows, use soap and water, rinse well, and squeegee dry. Your windows will shine like a new dime!

Instead of linoleum floor cleaner...

use white vinegar (about one cup per two gallons of water).

Instead of linoleum floor polish...

> use skim milk. (It doesn't smell, honest!)

Instead of air freshener...

> use herbal bouquets, pure vanilla on a cotton ball, or set out a
> bowl of simmered cinnamon sticks and whole cloves.

Instead of brass polish...

> make a paste of equal parts vinegar, salt, and flour. Be sure to
> rinse completely afterwards to prevent corrosion.

TROUBLE-FREE WHILE AWAKE AND ASLEEP

The solution to the dust problem in your living room and bedroom is a no-brainer: dust and vacuum regularly. Of course, I know you already do, but with the detoxification lifestyle you're adopting comes a new definition of the word "regularly." Once a day is by no means too often to take a dust mop to the floor and a dust rag to the furniture.

Since you're now cleaning for health instead of just neatness, you'll want to get under and behind the furniture. That's where the dust bunnies are, and they're feasts for dust mites. I'm not suggesting that you have somebody lift up the entertainment center for you to vacuum under every day, but you also don't want to wait months before cleaning up those hidden spots. I make it a point to rearrange my furniture on the slightest whim so I have an excuse to vacuum up the newly re-exposed rug area.

The same advice applies to your bedroom, where you should always vacuum under the bed.

Any time you vacuum, keep the room well ventilated. If your vacuum cleaner doesn't have a filter, get rid of it and get one that does. Wear a dust mask as you vacuum; there's a lot of dust, mold, and bacteria getting thrown into the air.

Wash your sheets, pillowcases, and blankets. All bedding should be washed in hot water twice a week. That's a lot of washing, but the alternative is lying in your own toxic waste dump, a gathering place for dead skin, dust mites, and bacteria. I usually recommend buying inexpensive blankets that you won't mind getting worn from the washing. If you have a very nice bedspread that you really can't have washed so often, fold it up and put it away while you sleep.

Cover your mattress and pillow for protection. You can find the appropriate protective material at stores specializing in helping people with asthma and allergies. Even if you don't have asthma or allergies, covering your mattress and pillows is a must for everybody. I urge you to take this step to clean up this part of your life right now. You probably spend about eight hours a day in that bed, at a time when your defenses are at their lowest. Some of my clients have had their VHI go up by as many as 15 points after they properly prepared their bedding and began to wash it more often.

Pack your pillowcase. I always carry along my own clean pillowcase and cover whenever I travel, since hotels treat their linen with intense chemical cleansers. When I failed to bring mine recently, I woke up the first morning not feeling adequately rested. The second morning I felt downright tired until I got up and moving. By the third day I was exhausted and by no means a happy camper! That night I simply wrapped the pillow in a freshly washed towel—and had no problems the next day.

LOVE YOUR PET . . . CLEANLY

Remember your mom telling you to wash your hands after you played with the household pet? Mom was right (as usual). Animals harbor a lot more parasites than humans—it's the nature of the beast. Just because you can't see them, doesn't mean those parasites aren't there. And just because you don't want to think about it doesn't mean cross-contamination hasn't transferred some of the pests to your own body.

So should you get rid of your pets? Of course not. But you can do lots of things to make sure your pet gives you love and loyalty, rather than toxicity.

Keep your pets out of the bedroom. The last thing you want is a parasite infestation in your bedding. You may cherish sharing your bed with your dog or cat, but be aware that you're exposing yourself to additional toxins that have a tendency to store themselves in your fat cells and plump those little babies up.

Give them their space. Ideally, there will be a specific room for your indoor pets. It should not be carpeted, since carpeting is an ideal breeding ground for parasites.

Wash their bedding regularly. Cat and dog dander, fleas and flea dirt, and germs from outdoors can accumulate quickly. Be diligent about washing your pets' own bedding. Wash and rinse in the hottest water you have.

Shampoo them once a week.

Schedule regular trips to the veterinarian. Take your pets to the vet regularly to make sure they are not harboring any unwanted pests. Have your pets "wormed" on a regular basis.

Cat-proof your air. There's no use denying that cats especially can be a health problem. Cats have a particular dander that is airborne and very toxic to the lungs, as much as cigarette smoke in some cases. I know very few households with cats where at least one family member isn't suffering from some kind of respiratory problems. It's usually one of the children. If you're going to have cats, *please* get free-standing air filters.

Cats are particularly cuddly little things and love to sleep with humans. Please do *not* let them sleep with your children; this could be causing all kinds of diffuse symptoms that you're unaware of. Children are still growing and developing and if that process is impeded early they could have lung, allergy, and gastrointestinal problems for literally the rest of their lives. If the cat has already established this night-time habit, then there are some steps you can take. Thoroughly clean and vacuum the room in question; wear a mask and keep the children away. If you can afford it, replace the child's old mattress with a new one. If not, vacuum the mattress then take it outside and leave it in the hot sun for a while. Purchase a good-quality mattress cover, one that zips closed, and a plastic box-spring cover. If you cannot afford a high-quality one, then get an inexpensive plastic one that zips closed, then lay a thick mattress pad on top of that. Get all the bedding taken care of first; otherwise you are being reinfected every time you sleep. Then look into a good parasite cleanse for everyone in the family. Take all the animals to the vet and have them wormed after the house has been cleaned, and then keep your pets in an area you know will have to have special cleaning.

PERSONAL HYGIENE WITH FEWER TOXINS

Here's an irony: The prevailing concept of a clean body in our society often requires toxic exposure in the form of chemical-laden products like deodorants, shampoos, and even soap. I'd never suggest that you sacrifice one iota of socially acceptable cleanliness. But there are some adjustments you can make to lighten the toxic exposure without feeling any less fresh or clean.

Change your toothbrush regularly. Don't wait for it to wear out. The idea is to use the brush to remove bacteria from your mouth, not reintroduce them! Get rid of that brush before its microbe population booms. I suggest changing it as a routine matter on the first of each month to help you remember.

In between, try soaking your toothbrush in one capful of either Everclear or 190-proof alcohol added to a cup of water. Change this mixture about once a week. You can also use this mixture as a sterilizing mouthwash. You can even add one half of a fresh lemon and gargle with that.

Limit your soap use. The less skin you allow to be covered with the thin film that soap leaves, the fewer toxins will be blocked from exiting your body. When showering, soap your private parts and under your arms, but scrub the rest of your body without soap (unless you're quite dirty, of course). When you do buy soap, choose the "natural" cleaning bars you find at health food stores. I use one made only of oatmeal and lilac.

Keep your own hair color. Would you eat or drink hair dye? Your scalp is one of the most vascular areas of your body, so applying hair dye is the equivalent of an intravenous injection. I believe that hairdressers with many years in the business have some significant health issues as a direct result of exposure to the toxic chemicals in hair dye. You've probably heard of the black lung disease suffered by coal miners who have spent years of their lives breathing coal dust. But have you heard about "white lung"? It refers to the state of hairdressers' lungs after breathing in the chemicals of cosmetology for so many years. With a decrease in the use of aerosols in recent years, white lung has thankfully become less of a problem. But the lesson it teaches us remains.

If your VHI is under 70, you shouldn't even walk into a hair salon.

If you choose to forge ahead, I just want you to associate how you feel afterwards. At least do a lemon push (see Chapter Six) before you go in and after you come out.

If you must color your hair, at least consider cutting down on the frequency of applications. You can have your hairdresser apply a "frosting" by putting a cap on you so the color doesn't touch your scalp. You can still breathe it, though, so cover your face with a towel when they lean you back to rinse it out. Insist they wash it very quickly to minimize your exposure.

If you apply your own color, switch to natural hair dyes from the health food store. Some are actually made from vegetables. Henna is another really nice way to go and is actually good for your hair. If you want brown or dark red you can use brewed tea or coffee, depending on the color and look you want.

Now for one of my more radical hair treatment suggestions: black strap molasses. I use it as a conditioner, but because my hair is blonde, it actually darkens my hair a shade or two. The best part is that the resulting shine and strength are unbelievable. If you want to try it, apply the molasses in the bath tub—the process can be very messy. But it's oh-so-rewarding. It will even replenish some of your skin nutrients.

Try alternative antiperspirants. Since your underarms are prime toxin absorbers, it's worth checking the health food stores for products that offer an alternative to applying toxic chemicals there. The aluminum in most commercially available antiperspirants has been linked to many things, Alzheimer's disease being the most prominent one. One good alternative is bile salts, sold under the brand name Tai.

Spend a little time, ask some questions, and try some products to see what works for you. Yes, this might be quite a change, but it's worth it.

Find a more chemical-free hair spray. No hair spray at all would be the best option. But as much as you might try avoid it, there might just be times when you really need your hair to behave. Again, get down to your health food store and experiment with natural hair sprays. Use a pump-delivered (rather than aerosol) spray. Step outside to spray your hair and try not to get any on your skin.

Use natural oils on your skin. Instead of rubbing in chemical-laden skin products and inviting them to take up residence in your cells, apply a very thin layer of olive oil, almond oil, or coconut oil immediately after you shower. Then pat yourself dry. It should be absorbed by the time you dress, sparing your clothes.

One of the best toxin-free skin-softening scrubs I've found is baking soda. Scrub it across your wet skin and you'll be soft as a baby's bottom all over when you finish. In the process, you'll be balancing the pH of your skin and helping exfoliation. Dry skin is simply an indication that we need to increase our good oil intake. Do that by taking a couple of tablespoons of flaxseed oil, or gel caps of omega-3 oils.

Use natural shampoos. This is an easy change in this day and age. Health food stores are overflowing with nontoxic shampoos made from natural substances. If you need motivation to change, take a look at the label of a typical commercial shampoo made from chemicals. The list of syllable-clogged toxic components is staggering. But also check the small type on the label of any other shampoo you buy. It's easy for companies to use natural-sounding names for a product loaded with chemical toxins. Especially avoid anything containing cetyl alcohol, and anything including the words laureth sulfate or lauryl sulfate.

YOUR EFFORTS WILL BE REWARDED

No toxic source is ever too small to avoid or protect yourself from. The cumulative effect of consistently eliminating even your minimal toxic will work wonders for you. The more you eliminate, the more you're aware of potential toxic exposure, so the task becomes easier over time. Ridding your body of toxins will become second nature. It will be your reward for your faithful nutraplenishing and for your efforts to detoxify.

In your garden. After hearing me chatter on about toxins everywhere you can just imagine what's in your dirt. The first spring I had my practice, it took me a couple of weeks to realize what was happening to all my clients. All of the sudden, most of my "sweet little ladies," as I call them, most in their sixties, started getting their arthritic symptoms back, their backs were hurting again, they were tired, etc. This was after many of them had been symptom-free for months, most having gotten off many prescription medications for pain. I have never gardened, so I didn't realize it was planting season. Finally, they all started talking about their aches and pains in one class, then switched to what each was planting for the season. Needless to say the ladies in that room made the connection as soon as I did.

There are literally hundreds of chemical fertilizers and pesticide products used in home gardening. Many of my ladies were using these chemicals and were working in soil that contained these chemicals from previous years. Not to mention the parasites, the mold, and the bacteria. I got them all back on track, but not without a lot of pain on their part.

If you must garden, keep the chemicals you use to a minimum. Please wear gloves and a mask when you work in the garden. Don't sit directly on the ground—use a small plastic stool or a kneeling pad. They'll keep you from direct contact with toxins in the soil. If you make a specific connection to gardening and feeling poorly, you may have to decide to get another hobby or alter this one to not being harmful.

One thing you're almost certain to be exposed to in your garden is mold. One of the largest resorts in the United States is right here in Nashville. They announced not long ago that their beautifully manicured golf course was closed—in peak season, so you know it had to be bad—because of a mold infestation. Please be very careful and take the precautions I recommend.

WATER, WATER, EVERYWHERE

An absolute necessity for your new detox lifestyle is to get into the habit of drinking lots of water every day. How does 128 ounces sound? Your ideal daily water intake is 1 ounce per pound of body weight. That's the equivalent of eight tall (16-oz.) glasses or sixteen regular (8-oz.) glasses, which I'm sure is more than you're used to. A lot more. I know that amount is really difficult to "swallow" right now, but if you build up gradually, you'll find that it's not hard to do.

Don't start chugging that much all at once if you're not used to it. You need to start with just a few extra sips and work your way up. Any new habit is difficult to begin because you have to think about it. But once you're in this habit, you'll never let it go again. My clients have been amazed over the years at how aware they become of their bodies' thirst after they get into the water-drinking habit.

And by water, I mean literally water. Not juice. Not iced tea. Not sports drinks (with their added sugars). And definitely not sodas—diet or otherwise. Just plain, pure, cell-healthy, toxin-busting water.

I don't want you to be part of the 75 percent of Americans who are chronically dehydrated. Your transformation from fat to lean depends on adequate hydration for a number of reasons.

Water flushes toxins from your body. Once you increase your water intake, your more frequent bathroom visits will remind you of water's role in the kidneys' processing of toxins for elimination through the urine. Just as important, though, is water's anticonstipation power. As you know, dietary fiber acts as a bulking agent, causing the stool to press against the colon wall, triggering the muscle contractions that create the urge to defecate. Without sufficient water, fiber won't swell up enough to get the job done. Water and fiber (along with exercise) are the keys to ending constipation and getting rid of toxins that have accumulated in the lower digestive tract.

Water encourages fat loss. Even mild dehydration will slow down your metabolism. So adequate water intake will help keep your body's metabolic fat-burning furnace stoked. More immediately, there is a direct connection between drinking more water and eating less. About a third of Americans have what's known as a weak thirst mechanism, which means they easily mistake thirst for hunger, with predictable unfortunate results. One study at the University of Washington found that a single glass of water shuts down late-night hunger pangs.

Water makes you feel better. Dehydration is a trigger of daytime fatigue, and a major cause of headaches. It's often the case that the water you take your aspirin with does more to relieve a headache than the pill itself. There's also growing evidence that just sixty-four ounces of water a day—half your goal—eases back and joint pain.

Keep It Clean

The last thing you want to do is pour 128 ounces of contaminated liquid into your body. After all, you're drinking water to flush toxins, not add them. That means tap water is out of the question, as economical as it may be. Many of the chemicals polluting our environment end up in the water supply, and then chlorine is added to kill micro-organisms.

The filtered water you buy at water machines (or filter yourself) can be acceptable, but not always. Your best bet for cleanliness is distilled water. There are other good bottled waters—I prefer Evian or Smart water. I understand, though, that your budget may be a concern when we're talking about going through five or so quarts a day. Just promise me you won't drink the water out of the faucet.

Keep It Going

The biggest challenge you'll have won't be buying bottled water but drinking so much of it. If you're typical, you're probably not used to drinking two regular-sized glasses of water every single day, let alone eight. So our water quota of 128 ounces really will be a lifestyle change. The biggest hurdle is deciding that you're going to make this adjustment. Then you can use a few tricks:

□ Carry a 32-ounce plastic bottle of water around with you and keep it at your desk or work station if you have one. Take some gulps whenever you look at the bottle or think about it. Finish off the bottle twice and you're halfway to your daily goal.

□ Make it a matter of routine to drink down a half a glass (4 oz.) before each meal, including mid-morning or mid-afternoon "mini-meals." If you also drink 4 more ounces immediately after, you've accumulated 40 ounces over five meals, about a third of your total. Keep going, you can do it!! Trust me, you will learn to love your water.

□ Drinking 8 ounces or more before your meal will get you closer to your goal, and it will also help you eat less. That can be good or bad. I found out years ago (during some really unhealthy eating years) that if I would just drink some water it would dilute my gastric juices and make my hunger pangs go away. Skipping meals entirely is not recommended, but we can all use this little trick to help us eat less to gain health and lose weight. But if you find that a premeal glass of water completely kills you're appetite, then don't drink as much.

□ Drinking lots of 4-ounce shots of water is the best hydration strategy if you can make it work for you. Most of the time you don't want to consume more than 4 ounces of water every thirty minutes. Any more than that races through you, pulling out toxins (good), but also carrying with it needed minerals called electrolytes (bad). That's the reason why you drink a lot of water all at once during the lemon pushes in your detox regime—that rush of water pushes things out of your system. But you don't want to be losing electrolytes many times a day.

☐ Try some of the fruit-flavored waters on the market to make the idea of so much water more appealing. Just be absolutely sure that there's no added sugar.

☐ If you're the type who craves carbonated drinks, substitute sparkling water with some lemon for one or two of your 16-ounce glasses in a day. This will help you wean yourself off soft drinks while helping you reach your water quota.

YOUR GOAL: PHARMACEUTICAL-FREE

Unlike the nutraceuticals that make up your nutraplenishing regimen, pharmaceuticals are chemicals. New drugs account for a good percentage of those two thousand synthetic chemicals introduced into the world every year. Almost all prescription and over-the-counter medications—from antidepressants to ibuprofen, from birth control pills to cortisone injections—fall into this category of synthetic chemicals.

That means pharmaceuticals are toxic. They are substances delivered to your system that don't belong there—the very definition of toxic. If you need proof, next time you pick up your prescription medicine, read through the required insert that describes your pharmaceutical's ingredients, actions, and side effects, and the cautions required. Whatever else they do, pharmaceuticals add to your toxic burden.

So should you stop taking your prescription medicine? *Absolutely not.* Should you work with your doctor to reduce your pharmaceutical intake, if possible, with an eye toward being pharmaceutical-free in the (healthier) future? Yes you should. Pharmaceuticals are not compatible with the detox lifestyle. They impede your progress from fat to lean. They are obstacles to your vibrant health.

But as you nutraplenish and detoxify, the symptoms that you're taking the pharmaceuticals for are more likely to disappear. As you begin to achieve your vibrant health, the pharmaceuticals may become unnecessary.

A client named Gay came to me at age thirty-six after her doctor told her she had to lose weight because of her dangerously high blood pressure. The only advice she got about how to do that was limited to the age-old standby of "eat right and exercise." Of course, she'd tried that many times with no permanent success. So she turned to us.

About three months after she started nutraplenishing, detoxing, and following the Nashville Diet, Gay visited her doctor again. What her doctor saw was a completely different young lady—four dress sizes smaller and glowing with health. When he took her blood pressure, he thought the pressure cuff was broken. He left the room and came back with another one, took her blood pressure again, and got an even lower reading. Gay told us later she couldn't help but laugh, knowing that the surprised doctor would have to not just lower her blood pressure medication, but take her off it completely.

That's the kind of result you can achieve if you're faithful to your nutrient and detox regimens. Vibrant health is a pharmaceutical's worst enemy.

THE GOOD, THE BAD, AND THE EXCESS

I'm a pharmacist. I've seen the amazing good that pharmaceuticals can accomplish. Pharmaceuticals can save lives. They can relieve misery. They can eliminate symptoms. Many of my clients absolutely need prescription medications when they first come in. I'm the first to acknowledge that some toxicity is a small price to pay for the miracles that medicinal drugs can do.

But I've also seen the harm pharmaceuticals can do. I've seen them overprescribed. I've seen them used to alleviate symptoms while doing nothing about the real condition causing those symptoms. I've seen how the "cure" is slowly killing us.

I myself used to be part of the problem. When I worked at VA hospitals as a staff pharmacist in Texas and Tennessee, I would send those poor veterans away with grocery sacks full of prescription medication. I'd stand

and watch them with tears in my eyes as they walked off in their drugged torpor. Later, when I became more aware of the harm these drugs were inflicting, I'd start my own little education campaign with pharmacy customers, using a yellow highlighter to point out harmful side effects and talking to them about their eating habits and alternatives to pharmaceuticals. The store owners weren't always happy with me for that, as you can imagine.

Still, the sheer number of prescription drugs that so many people are on is frightening. Most of my clients have weight problems that are directly connected with chronic fatigue syndrome, fibromyalgia, prescription medication, mold, or parasite infestation, or combinations and — in extreme cases (VHI in the 30s and below)—all of the above. But, remember we tackle things one at a time in bite-size amounts. Most of them are taking no fewer than seven prescription medications: antianxiety pills such as Xanax, antidepressants like Prozac, pain medications, sleeping pills, cortisone injections, anti-inflammatories, and muscle relaxers. Maybe a case can be made for taking any one of those drugs for a brief period. But being on all seven at once long-term isn't going to make anybody healthy.

The sad part is that so many of these toxic drugs deal only with the symptoms and not the condition causing those symptoms. Sure, it's nice to be able to dance the night away because your pain is being numbed by a drug, but what's that doing to improve your health? Nothing.

Pain is a message that something's wrong, like the oil light on your car. What do you do when that oil light comes on? Take out the little bulb so it will go off? Hello!!? You change the oil! You do what needs to be done to help the car run better. And then, you know what? That light will go out.

Doctors resort to pharmaceuticals not because they don't care, or because they're greedy. I don't agree with those in "alternative" medicine who question the motives of the medical establishment. I've worked with physicians most of my life and I've never met one who wasn't firmly dedicated to helping his or her patients. But the fact is that doctors rely on the pharmaceutical approach because that's what they know. That's how they were trained, and that's how they practice.

There was a time during my illness when I spent more than $900 a month on prescription medications. I didn't get better. Only after I discovered nutraceuticals and the importance of detoxification was I able to find a better way to health. Once I started to work with my body's natural healing capacity, nourishing it by nutraplenishing and clearing it of toxins, I was able to wean myself off pharmaceuticals, regaining my vibrant health and old dress size in the process—not to mention saving $900 a month. As I write this I've been pharmaceutical-free for four years. I want you to be as well.

WEANING YOURSELF OFF PRESCRIPTION DRUGS

Even though your nutraplenishing and detox regimens can improve your health enough to make it possible to quit pharmaceuticals, the impetus for actually eliminating prescription drugs from your life must come from you. That alone is a big step, since you may never even have thought about getting off pharmaceuticals until you started reading this chapter. Once you decide that vibrant health is preferable to a prescription drug regimen, there are some steps you can take to begin the transition. As with everything in the Nashville Diet, go slowly, one step at a time.

Don't just stop taking your prescription medicine. Under no circumstances should you act on your own to get off pharmaceuticals. You must not change anything that has to do with your drug regimen without your doctor's knowledge and approval.

Work with your doctor. Weaning yourself off pharmaceuticals must be a cooperative effort between you and your physician. The suggestion may have to come from you, but the implementation is your prescribing doctor's decision. You are the expert on how you feel, the status of your symptoms, and what you ultimately want; he or she is the expert on the drug's properties, consequences of a lower dose, and the conditions that must be met to change the prescription.

Inform your doctor about your supplementation program. This is important from the very beginning, even if you're not looking to eliminate prescription medications. Again, if you're on prescription medications, talk to your doctor before starting your nutraplenishing regimen. The person who's treating you and prescribing drugs for you needs to be aware of what else you're putting into your body, even beneficial nutrients. When you're ready to get off pharmaceuticals, most doctors encourage your determination to improve your own health. Even if they're skeptical about the benefits of supplementation, most doctors will try to work with you on reducing your pharmaceutical dosages if they consider it a safe course.

And while the pharmaceutical companies might not like the idea of nobody at all taking pharmaceuticals, I believe that your doctor would love to see you become pharmaceutical-free.

Nutraplenish first. Here again, the Nashville Diet approach applies—that is, renourish your system through nutraceuticals and reduce your toxic burden so your entire body is stronger and healthier overall. Only then does eliminating your prescription medication become a possibility. Remember, nutraceuticals do not replace pharmaceuticals. They don't treat disease. But they do restore your body's ability to heal itself. Give them time. Nutraplenish for at least sixty days and detoxify for thirty days before approaching your doctor about relief from your medications.

Eliminate one drug at a time. Unless your doctor tells you differently, I recommend eliminating one pharmaceutical at a time. The task, like any other you undertake on the Nashville Diet, is more manageable in bite-size chunks. Also, if you experience setbacks as you wean yourself from drugs, you'll be better able to pinpoint the cause.

Taper off little by little. Cold turkey usually isn't the best way to quit a prescription drug. In some cases your doctor may take you off a pharmaceutical completely and see what happens, but it's generally preferable to slowly reduce the dosage and monitor the results.

YOU AND YOUR JOURNAL

Your quest to recover your best weight and overall health surely qualifies as one of the great journeys of your life. Don't you want to write it down? I require all my clients to keep a journal. I want you to do it, too.

The journal I want you to keep is not the typical "food journal" that many diets urge. I don't want you to count calories or fat grams or every millisecond you spend on a treadmill, and then fill up your journal with those numbers until it looks like an algebra textbook.

Keep track of your nutrients. It's important that you keep track of your nutrient regimen. Whether you do it in your journal or tack it to your wall, you need to keep precise count of what nutrients you're taking, the doses, and when you take them. Any adjustments in your regimen should be carefully noted. Consistency is the key with your nutrients, and this is the only way to ensure that consistency.

Keep track of your feelings. In addition to tracking your nutrient regimen, it's important that you record in your journal how you feel. Write down how you're feeling emotionally, spiritually, and physically each day, or at various times of the day. You can do this any way you want—with short notes or expanded poetry. It's your journal, so write whatever you want in any way you want.

But do include the foods you eat each day. You don't need to break this down into fine detail, or chart it out by time of day (although you may if you want). General terms will do. A typical early entry might read like this: "This morning I ate my usual fried eggs with toast, but I had one egg instead of two. It seemed strange not having that second egg on my plate, but I felt just as full afterwards. Later in the morning I felt like lying down at the usual time."

Another important "feeling" to include is any food cravings you might have. Get those nagging cravings out of the deep recesses of your mind and onto paper. When do they seem worse? When do they let up? What foods do you crave? Do you crave different foods at different times of day? Write it down!

One goal of such a journal is to make connections between what you eat and how you feel. Over time, you'll start to detect patterns and eventually be able to pin down your problem foods and see the kinds of results that occur over time with diet changes. But the most valuable payoff of everyday journaling is the way it keeps you focused on your noble mission. You'll find that the very act of writing in your journal gives you encouragement and keeps you moving in the right direction. A journal engages you in your own health, your own life.

This goes to the heart of the matter. When you chose to embark on the Nashville Diet, you made more than a decision to lose fat and gain energy. You decided, perhaps for the first time, to take charge of your own health. You decided to take that control away from cravings, from chemicals, and from diet doctors. You know that the power to overcome your weight and health problems lies within you. That's why you're going to succeed!

Moving on:

exercise that works in the real world

"diet and exercise" is the mantra we've all heard for just about every approach to weight loss over the last several decades. Where has it gotten us today? Not far. More people are more overweight than ever.

The mantra of the Nashville Diet is *not* "diet and exercise." It is "nutraplenishing and detoxification." I don't believe in starving and stairclimbing yourself into leanness. I believe in reversing the health-related factors that lead to weight gain in the first place. After you renourish your cells and flush accumulated toxins out of them, you can easily and naturally adjust the way you eat and get your body in motion to achieve your ideal weight and stay there.

Of course, that doesn't mean that "diet and exercise" don't enter into the picture. They most assuredly do. I'll be giving you plenty of help and guidelines for developing healthy and satisfying eating habits (that's coming up in Part Three). And starting right now, I'll be urging you to do yourself a favor by adding a little exercise into your life.

Now, I'm well aware that this may not be the most welcome of news. Many of my clients moan with dread the first time I mention the E word.

And no wonder. They're lethargic from years of being overweight, under-nourished, and in poor health, and often suffer from fibromyalgia or chronic fatigue syndrome. Since I've been where they are, I can understand why bed seems more appealing to them than a brisk walk.

But you know what? That's exactly the reason it's so important to start exercising as soon as your nutraplenishing has lifted your VHI enough to do it. Your body was made to move. And it isn't happy unless it does. Exercise is one of the four essential components of vibrant health (along with cellular rebuilding through nutraplenishing, detoxification, and proper nutrition). Since all four components are integrated and enhance each other, exercise speeds your progress from fat to lean.

In fact, exercise works in conjunction with the rest of your fat-to-lean strategies in two key ways. One, it benefits your body at the cellular level, promoting detoxification of your fat cells and smoother functioning of your detoxification pathways, such as your immune and lymphatic systems. That's why rebounding, an especially effective cellular exercise, is included in your detox regimen.

Two, exercise boosts your metabolic rate—that is, the efficiency with which your body processes food into energy. Keeping your metabolic furnace burning is a central strategy of the Nashville Diet. Exercise helps the cause by building lean muscle mass, which is active tissue that requires energy to stay alive. Lean muscle mass burns calories throughout the day—not just when you're exercising—and works to break down fat cells.

Put Your Fat Uniform to Better Use

When my weight was high and my health was low, I wore what I called my "fibromyalgia-fat uniform" pretty much every day. You know the outfit, don't you? A loose t-shirt, sweat pants, and shoes you can kick off or slip on in a millisecond. This "uniform" allowed me to spend most of my time in bed, and not have to use energy to change out of pajamas on the rare occasion I ventured out into the world.

I wasn't the only woman in the nation to don that uniform daily. And it's still a fashion statement among the overweight today, especially those who are so constantly fatigued or pained that they rarely leave their beds. Look around on the streets and you'll see that uniform on lots of women and men. Perhaps you need only look in the mirror.

The fat uniform may be comfortable, but what a sad statement that its wearer has too little energy to even try to look good, let alone lead a fulfilling life. The good news is that nutraplenishing will lift you to the point where you can do something about your inactive condition. But it won't happen automatically. It's up to you to shake out the cobwebs and take action and start exercising.

Unlike others, you have the advantage of a nutraplenishing regimen to get you ready for exercise. And if you've been wearing a fat uniform, you have another advantage. Lace up a pair of sneakers to go with it and you've got a perfectly functional exercise outfit.

TEN MORE REASONS TO EXERCISE

I haven't met too many people who didn't enjoy exercise once they got into it. The trick is to gather up enough motivation to stick with it for the first few weeks. After that, you'll be in love with the joy of moving and the noticeable benefits it delivers.

With a little introspection, you may discover your own personal sources of motivation. As a health care professional, I think the undeniable benefits of exercise should be sufficient motivation. If the detox and metabolic benefits I've already described aren't enough for you, here are some more facts to pique your interest in exercise:

1. **Exercise improves your overall health.** Study after study has confirmed this, using such health indicators as oxygen uptake efficiency, the ratio of lean tissue to fat, cardiovascular functioning, and so on.

2. **Exercise helps protect you from disease.** High blood pressure, osteoporosis, heart disease, cancer, and diabetes are less likely in exercisers than in sedentary people. On a day-to-day level, one recent

study showed that those who exercise just twenty minutes a day twice a week are significantly less likely to call in sick to work than nonexercisers.

3. Exercise relieves your stress. Hormones known as endorphins are released through exercise and act as a natural hormone balancer to reduce stress. That's why so many exercisers testify to feeling more at peace during and after exercise.

4. Exercise improves your figure. The combination of muscle toning and fat loss from exercise works miracles. For example, abdominal exercises have been called "the natural tummy tuck."

5. Exercise clears your mind. After just a few weeks on a steady exercise schedule, you'll notice that the "fog" has lifted, you're thinking more clearly, and decisions are easier to make.

6. Exercise boosts your self-esteem. This is a tremendous and unexpected benefit of exercise for many people. This particular side effect creates a self-perpetuating positive cycle, because your increased confidence allows you to do even more, thus boosting your self-esteem further.

7. Exercise reduces your risk of injury. Toned muscles take the strain off injury-prone joints, and the strength they bring makes mishaps less likely. Furthermore, stronger bones from exercise are better able to withstand bumps and falls.

8. Exercise gives you more energy. A healthier heart and stronger lungs are direct results of exercise. Combine those benefits with less fat and more muscle, and you're rarin' to go.

9. Exercise keeps you alive. The connection between regular exercise and longevity has been firmly established. As many as 250,000 deaths per year in the United States alone have been attributed to a lack of physical activity.

10. Exercise keeps you looking younger. Now, who wouldn't want that?

BEFORE YOU START

Wouldn't it be great if that list of nutraplenishing supplements I gave you included an "exercise pill" that would bring you the benefits of exercise with one swallow a day? No such luck, I'm afraid. But you do have the next best thing—a whole regimen of capsules that are nourishing your cells in such a way that you can work *with* your body as you begin to exercise, instead of against it.

If you've never been able to "get up" for exercise before—or if you've tried and quickly given it up—your nutraplenishing program represents a new opportunity. It will put you on the launching pad where your exercise efforts can really take off.

So take care of first things first. Give the nutrients time to prepare your body for taking that next step into exercise. If you're already exercising, by all means continue doing so as you work your way through the first stages of nutraplenishing and detoxification. If you're newcomer to exercise, I've got a few more guidelines for you:

- ☐ Follow your nutraplenishing program for at least a month before starting in on exercise.
- ☐ If completing the three-week detox regimen (described in Chapter Six) while simultaneously starting an exercise program is an overwhelming task for you, do the detox first.
- ☐ Your VHI should be at least 70 before you begin your exercise program.
- ☐ Consult your doctor before embarking on any exercise program, especially if you've been chronically ill.

JUST MAKE THE FIRST MOVE

This is not an exercise book. I won't burden you with complex or demanding workout regimens. What I will give you is a simple and realistic plan to gain the health and weight-loss benefits of exercise. You don't even have to think of what I'm recommending as exercise; think of it as simply getting moving again.

The biggest step you'll take in your exercise efforts is that first one out of bed or off the couch. I did my first "sit-up"—meaning I actually started my exercise program—by sitting up in bed and staying that way for thirty-minute increments. After starting the nutrient regimen, I would sit up . . . and then *get* up. A major step forward! Just standing up to take a shower was, for me, exercise at the time, since I hadn't had the strength to stand up long enough to take a shower for over two years. Then I started walking "laps" around the bedroom. Eventually I graduated to laps around the whole house. Then one day my fourteen-year-old daughter came home from school and found me sitting in the front of the house. I had actually walked five houses down and back. With tears in her eyes she said to me, "Mom, now we have hope." And she was absolutely right.

But we had more than hope. I had started something that would get me my health and fit body back. And so can you. Now, some five years later, I can do sit-ups until I get bored, twenty military pushups, and run for a couple of miles. So when it's time for you to get moving, go for it— even if you have to start with just sitting up, getting up, and walking around inside the house.

To take that first step from sedentary to active, the most important body part to focus on is your mind. Don't listen to those old tapes in your head that are saying you're lazy or unmotivated. That's not what's been going on. You had no "gas" to get up and do anything until now. What's changed? You're building your system back by nutraplenishing and detox-ifying. Now you're ready to embrace the good news that physical activity— your body in motion—is something to seek rather than avoid. Perhaps you've already understood your body's desire for movement from the tai chi and rebounding in the detox regimen.

If not, here's a suggestion. Ease yourself into exercising by spending ten to twenty minutes a day five days a week doing an invigorating "nonex-ercise" that you enjoy—such as gardening, practicing the tai chi that you're now familiar with, playing with children, or participating in a light sport like Ping-Pong, badminton, or Frisbee.

Another great way to ease into physical activity is to impose a little bit of extra effort on yourself during your typical day. Take stairs instead of elevators or escalators. Park farther away so you can walk a bit. Rake the leaves yourself. (Be sure to wear a mask and gloves when you do; mold, mildew, parasites, and many other toxins live on those leaves and dirt.) Wash your own car. Yes, you've probably spent most of your life trying to get out of doing those very things. Now do your body a favor by working them into your schedule. A warning, though: These little ploys for sneaking in exercise are so popular these days that you may find the stairs crowded and all the far-away parking spaces taken.

EXERCISE YOUR WAY TO VIBRANT HEALTH

Once you've gotten used to the feeling of extra physical activity, you're ready move on to a more structured routine. That's when you'll really start feeling the benefits.

So what do I mean when I talk about "exercise"? Two things. The first is cardiovascular exercise, sometimes called aerobic exercise, but now usually shortened to "cardio." This type of exercise requires you to keep up a physical activity over a period of time as you steadily breathe in oxygen to burn calories to fuel your effort. The two biggest benefits of cardio are fat loss and improved heart health.

The other exercise category is strength training, which builds and tones your muscles. This is more properly called resistance training, because it forces your muscles to work against something that's resisting their effort. That something can be a weight (like a dumbbell) but it doesn't have to be. Although strength training's main benefit is improved muscle tone (and the welcome extra strength that goes with it), it also complements your fat-to-lean efforts because the added lean muscle mass it gives you serves to boost your metabolic rate. That translates into more fat burning during the twenty-three and a half hours of the day you're not exercising.

As a beginner, plan on dedicating twenty minutes a day to cardiovascular exercise, three to five times a week. Allot about fifteen minutes two to three days a week for your strength-training work. That comes to only about two hours of the one hundred and sixty-eight hours in a week.

Not too high a price to pay for all those fat-to-lean and vibrant health benefits, I'd say.

Schedule your exercise session before meal time. That way, the elevated blood sugar levels induced by your exercise will curb your appetite at the table. This trick also gives your system the tools to actually use the incoming food as fuel rather than store it as fat or cellulite. But let at least ten minutes pass after a workout before you eat.

CARDIO EXERCISE

Any heart-pumping activity that you can maintain for at least twelve minutes at a time makes for a fine cardio workout. The most popular cardio exercises are jogging, cycling, and swimming. If you join a health club or have some money to spend on home equipment, you also have the options of a treadmill, an exercise bike, a stair-climber, a cross-country ski machine, or a number of other ergonomically designed exercise machines.

Which is best? The experts usually answer that question by saying, "whatever you enjoy the most." It's a good answer, because what matters most is that you work hard enough to elevate your heart rate, that you keep going for at least twelve minutes (working your way up to twenty or more over time), and that you do it at least three days a week. You're more likely to accomplish all those things if you're doing something you enjoy.

In my experience, however, people who aren't used to exercising don't enjoy any of those options. If that's you, I have two recommendations for a beginning cardio program:

Walking

Good, old-fashioned walking is way under-rated as a cardiovascular exercise. I'm convinced that we'd have a healthier world if everybody would just get out there and walk. If you're new to exercise, I can't think of a better way to get started than to go out the door and start walking.

Let me make a confession. I've never been an eager-beaver exerciser. For many years I was so sick and fatigued that exercise was out of the question. Then, after I discovered nutraplenishing, I was so busy researching and counseling others that I neglected my own advice, to walk, that is. But there came a time when I knew I needed to do something physical, so I decided to get into walking.

With my first experience in walking, as I've already admitted, I didn't go much farther than my mail box. But even making it to a house down the block was a big deal for me, having spent so much time barely able to walk around my bedroom. I added two houses per day until I got to the point where I could walk up and down the hills in my neighborhood for two miles.

I began to love it. I loved the exhilaration of my body in motion. I loved spending that time walking with a girlfriend or alone with my thoughts. I loved that satisfied feeling of making it back home tired but at the same time energized by the workout.

Then I started to pick up the pace to get more of the cardiovascular benefits—that is, a stronger heart, improved circulation, and more lung power. After a brisk pace started feeling comfortable, I slowly worked a little jogging into my walks. I enjoyed the extra challenge so much that I set a goal of being able to jog to the top of a not-so-nearby hill. It took me six weeks to reach that goal, but let me tell you the first time I made it up I felt like Rocky at the top of those steps.

If you think walking might be your best path to an exercise program, follow in my footsteps. It's just a matter of some simple steps:

- ☐ Get some comfortable walking shoes or sneakers. It's the only equipment you need.
- ☐ Decide on a good time of day for you to take your walk, and then walk at that time five or six times a week.
- ☐ At first, don't worry about how far or fast you go. Just focus on faithfully getting out there every day until you're in the habit.
- ☐ Work your way up so you're walking at least fifteen minutes out and fifteen minutes back, for a total of half an hour.

- Once you can comfortably put in half an hour five days a week, start concentrating on picking up your pace. Don't worry about complicated formulas for reaching your "training zone." When you're walking briskly enough for a half hour to get true cardio benefits, you'll know it.
- Incorporate intervals of jogging into your walk when you're ready to. Don't force it. One of these days it will just seem like a good idea to jog a block or two. Next thing you know, you're off and running!
- Enjoy yourself. Walking is natural, healthy, and fun. It's a beautiful world out there. Appreciate it!

Rebounding

The same activity I gave you in the last chapter as a detox technique is also a wonderful mode of cardiovascular exercise. So since you're doing it anyway, why not kill several birds with one stone? You'll be improving the health of your cells, speeding up the elimination of toxins from your body, expanding your heart and lung capacity, burning calories, boosting your metabolic rate, and even strengthening your lower body and midsection. All this from bouncing up and down on an undersized trampoline!

If you choose rebounding as your cardio mode, it's a simple matter to convert it from a mostly cellular exercise to an aerobic one. Do the following:

- Jump for at least twenty minutes, five times a week. If you're beginning, work your way up to that schedule, both in minutes and days. Use my rebounding instructions in Chapter Six as a guide.
- Do the shallow, feet-touching bounce for the first few minutes of your session as a warm-up.
- Vary the initial "health bounce" stage of your workout: (1) Tap one heel in front of you as you bounce with the

other, then switch; (2) lift one heel behind you toward your buttocks as you bounce with the other leg, knee slightly bent, then do the same with the opposite leg; (3) reach back and tap your heel with your hand as you do the heel-to-buttock variation.

□ Let your feet leave the surface with each bounce for the rest of your session but just slightly.

□ Concentrate on pushing down on the surface with the balls of your feet as you land rather than on jumping up.

□ Jog in place, run in place, or otherwise alternate your feet for half the remaining time. But unlike the aerobic bounce in the detox regimen, let one foot come up just a tad from the surface with each step.

□ Vary your aerobic bounce: Place your arms straight and twist from the waist down as you jog or punch diagonally as you keep your body forward.

□ Fill the remaining time with strength bouncing, springing straight up and down with your feet together, your knees slightly bent and your hands out for balance.

□ Vary your strength bounce: Bring your arms parallel to the ground at your sides and then down to your sides as you bounce.

These are, of course, vary basic guidelines. If you stick with rebounding long enough, you'll want to look for a good book (yes, there are books on rebounding) or a trainer to bring new challenges to your rebounding routine.

STRENGTH TRAINING

The health and appearance benefits of strength training are so well recognized these days that you'll find men and women of all shapes and ages in fitness centers anywhere in the country. One way you can begin your strength training is to join a health club and have one of the staff instructors get you started on a beginning program.

Another option is to invest in some home exercise equipment—either light barbells and a bench, or a multi-purpose exercise machine. Then book some sessions with a personal trainer so you'll learn how to put the equipment to good use and use it properly.

But if you've never done a strength exercise in your life, I recommend testing the waters with a simple, at-home routine that requires no equipment whatsoever. Instead of using weights, the resistance will come from your own body weight working against gravity.

The following three exercises combine to tone muscles in your upper body, your lower body, and your midsection. Do them two days a week at first, then three. The secret to success is quality, not quantity. So pay more attention to doing the movements as described than to just getting them done. I'd rather see you do one crunch right than one hundred wrong.

Crunches

These are better than sit-ups because they don't put unnecessary stress on your back. They'll strengthen your midsection, especially the abdominal muscles covering your tummy.

- ☐ Lie on your back with your knees bent, feet flat, and spine flush to the floor. Place all ten fingers lightly at the back of your head, elbows out.
- ☐ Position your chin as if it were holding an orange and find a focus spot on the ceiling.
- ☐ Tighten your stomach area as you bring your upper torso up, letting your chin move toward the ceiling until your shoulders, but not your lower back, are off the floor.
- ☐ Focus on your abdominal muscles doing the work as you come up.
- ☐ Come back down slowly and in control.

☐ Try to do five the first time (it might seem like a lot) and work your way up to twenty-five at a time.

Pushups

A great all-around upper-body exercise! Push-ups will strengthen your chest and upper back muscles as well as your arms and shoulders. This exercise, if done military style, will focus on the upper body yet use every muscle in the body.

☐ Lie face down with your palms flat on the floor on either side of your head, slightly wider than shoulder-width apart. Your body should be in a straight line from your heads to your toes.

☐ Simply push your upper body up so your arms straighten, your toes supporting your lower body.

☐ Hold at the top for a beat and keep your body straight as you lower back down slowly and in control. Stop just before your chest hits the floor and start the next one.

☐ Begin with one and work up first to twelve and then to twenty.

☐ You may find you have trouble doing even one at first. No problem. Keep everything the same, but support your lower body with your knees instead of your toes. You'll still find the movement challenging, but more doable.

Squats

It's not the most pleasant of names for an exercise, but this one will do wonders for your entire lower body, from your calves to your buttocks.

☐ Stand with feet shoulder-width apart, knees slightly bent. Hold your arms out in front of you, or put one hand on something solid like a desk top for support.

☐ Bend your knees and keep your back straight and abdominal muscles tight as you lower yourself down until your upper thighs are parallel to the floor, almost like sitting back into a chair.

☐ Push your feet into the floor and squeeze the muscles in your buttocks as you bring yourself back up.

☐ Balance will be a problem at first, and you probably won't make it all the way down. Patience and persistence are the answer.

☐ Begin with five and work up to twelve, then twenty.

ANY LAST DOUBTS?

Just these three strength exercises—crunches, pushups, and squats—will fast-forward your fat-to-lean project as long as you practice them regularly. These can be done anywhere, too. If you're like many of my clients, though, you may still harbor some doubts about the whole idea of strength training. Here are some typical concerns—and my answers.

"**Won't I get too muscled up and bulky?**" I don't like the way bodybuilders look. Those men and women dedicate most of their waking hours to intense heavy lifting to get that way. You're not doing anything like that.

"**Still, won't strength training make me bigger? I'm trying to get smaller!**" You're trying to lose fat. More muscle mass helps you do that. So the end result is you'll be trimmer and shapelier from strength training.

"**Why am I bothering with upper body exercises? Shouldn't I do more exercises for my thighs? That's where most of my fat is.**" Where you build muscle has nothing to do with where you lose fat. It's healthiest to strengthen all your major muscle groups. Your body will lose fat according to its own genetic patterns. You can't "spot-reduce."

"If these exercises help me lose weight, why don't I do them every day?" You do resistance exercise to make your muscles work harder than they're used to. As they recover from the exercise, they adapt to the additional stress they've been through by coming back bigger and stronger than they were before. So it's important to give them enough recovery time between exercise sessions, so they can finish building up before you break them down again. Instead of doing strength training more often, look to add more intensity to the workouts you already do. How? When you're ready, use a personal trainer or one of the many fine strength-training books available to add new exercises to your repertoire, using dumbbells or exercise machines. You'll love the added results.

3

ACHIEVE YOUR
VIBRANT HEALTH

THE PROBLEM:

craving to eat, eating to crave

one of the things I love most about my job is that I travel around the country a great deal—helping clients, promoting my clinic, scouting suppliers, and doing research. And although I love the travel, the flights can be long and tedious, so I'm always looking for ways to make good use of the time. As I was working on the manuscript for this book, I found myself on a long flight to Arizona to help a client who was too sick and overweight to make it to Nashville.

I decided to pass the time by sizing up my fellow passengers. How many, I wondered, had their vibrant health? How many on that plane were not overweight, looked like they were feeling strong and energetic, showed a glowing complexion, had healthy hair and nails, and seemed happy, with a relaxed demeanor free of stress and anger? The plane was full, and I walked slowly down the aisle to check out every single passenger. Know how many winners I found? Two. And one of them, it turned out, was a twenty-year-old young lady who had been taking hard drugs for years and was now on Prozac. Since you don't have your vibrant health if you're on prescription medication, she had to be disqualified. That left one person out of 200 or so with vibrant health. Yours truly.

You can't imagine how discouraging such an observation can be for a health professional. The statistics that tell us that three out of four Americans are overweight are shocking enough. But they're nothing compared to the discovery that you can surround yourself with hundreds of average Americans and not one of them is truly healthy.

All this was sinking in when the other shoe dropped. The flight attendants started handing out snack boxes, leading to a chilling scene that I'll never forget. Every single person on that plane started tearing into those snacks with reckless abandon, as though they hadn't eaten in weeks. And what was this "food" they were so desperately gulping? Over-processed, chemical-laden, toxin-rich, nutritionally worthless cookies, "cheese" crackers, and candy. And of course there were complimentary soft drinks to wash it all down. I realized I was watching a planeload of unhealthy people voluntarily poisoning themselves. I felt like standing up and yelling, "Stop! All of you! Can't you see what you're doing? You're taking poison! Please don't do it!"

I didn't, of course, but the message those passengers would have heard from me was and is the literal truth. Americans are poisoning themselves with the way they eat, and that's why most of them are sluggish, unhealthy, and overweight. The gusto with which those people on the plane went after those nutritionally worthless and health-harming snacks confirmed in a very human way the message that my research and experience had taught me.

Cravings dictate the eating habits of most people. You've heard of Thoreau's famous observation that many people "lead lives of quiet desperation." Well, that pretty much describes the nutritional lives of most Americans. Their imbalanced systems drive them to eat not just too much food, but too much of the wrong foods. Those wrong foods lead to more imbalance, and the cycle continues as the fat accumulates and the clothes sizes go up and up.

THE RIGHT STUFF

There's a sequel to the airplane story. At the hotel I stayed at I noticed a sweet young couple with three children, the oldest not more than five years old. I watched all five of them eat breakfast from the small buffet table four days in a row. For four straight mornings, they ate waffles, muffins, toast, bacon, and sausages, with coffee and some alleged juice that was more sugar and additives than anything that had ever known a fruit tree. It broke my heart to see such a lovely family treating their bodies this way. What would that young man and woman look and feel like five years from now? What kind of future did the children have to look forward to? The sadness of the sight brought home two lessons about our eating habits today and why so many people are struggling with their weight. One was the undeniable fact that that family really didn't have much of a choice at that buffet table other than various forms of refined flour and sugar and processed meat carefully chosen for maximum levels of saturated fat and cholesterol. That's the sad truth of today's society. Unhealthy food is the norm. We are surrounded by it, bombarded with it, and constantly urged to buy and eat more of it. It truly takes a proactive effort to free yourself from it.

The other point here is that this young couple had no inkling that any such effort was needed. They didn't have the slightest clue that they were jeopardizing their long-term health and eating their way to obesity. After all, in their minds, they were simply partaking of a typical American breakfast. Most people are tragically unaware that it's the kind of food they eat, not just the amount they eat, that is causing their health and weight problems.

You are no longer one of those people. By nutraplenishing and detoxifying, you're eliminating the cravings for too much of the wrong foods. You're preparing your body for fat loss as you begin to eat the right amount of food to meet your body's needs and keep you satisfied. You will replace problem foods with good foods. You will stop eating too much of the wrong stuff and start eating healthy amounts of the right stuff. Not just while you're "on a diet," but forever. No sacrifice. No cravings. No quiet desperation. No feelings of deprivation. Just good, healthy eating so you can get on with the rest of your life.

Unlike my fellow airline passengers and that nice family in the hotel, you will understand the difference between harmful food and healthy food. And unlike them, you will eventually be able to make a smooth transition from one to the other. Why? Because your nutraplenishing regimen and detox efforts will restore enough balance to your system to enable you to break the craving cycle that's been imprisoning you in a life of low energy and high weight.

PROBLEM FOODS: IDENTIFYING THE CULPRITS

It's no oversimplification to say that you're overweight today because you've been eating too much of the wrong foods. But *why* you've been eating too much of the wrong foods is where it gets more complicated. We've been looking at the "whys" of the matter throughout this book.

One thing's for sure, though. It's not because you've been making poor food choices. The truth is, you've had very little choice in the matter. The nutritional deficiencies and the resulting craving cycles and imbalances pretty much doom you to "quick-fix" foods that satisfy the cravings . . . for a while. And because of the nature of our food supply, those quick-fix foods not only tend to lack nutrients, they're usually loaded with toxins, chemicals, and other unhealthy contents that exacerbate your weight and health problems. Obviously, this has got to stop. I've found that it's most helpful to first make clear just what the worst of the "problem foods" are. Most of my clients find the list eye-opening, to say the least. You might too.

PREPACKAGED AND PROCESSED FOODS

This is a huge category of unhealthy food that most people eat regularly without giving it a second thought. I'm not exaggerating in the slightest when I tell you that the national love affair with processed foods is destroying the health of America. If you do nothing else than eliminate these impostors from your diet, you'll have made a huge leap from fat to lean.

My definition of processed food is simple: It's any food that's been altered so it can be packaged, stored, prepared, and eaten with maximum "convenience." Most of the time, that means whatever nutritive value there may have been in the original food has been replaced by any number of the hundreds of synthetic chemicals that are approved as food additives.

As a seasoned label reader, you'll find yourself constantly shocked at the way ingredients we recognize as food are lost amid a sea of synthetics that only a trained chemist could identify. Even the flavors are artificial. The same rules that apply to reading food labels apply to nutraceuticals. We've been taught to go by the Nutrition Facts panel. But the Nutrition Facts panel has no bearing on what ingredients are actually in the product. Remember, we eat food! We no longer take synthetic chemicals in our supplements and we certainly don't want to eat them either.

What's more, creations (I hate to call them food) that have been packaged and processed are notorious for going heavy on the very same problem foods I'm warning you about—sugar, salt, refined flour, bad fats and so on. Check out the label on just about any ready-made dessert or even a commercial cereal and you'll see what I mean.

FROZEN YOGURT

Nutrition Facts
Serving Size 1 Tbsp (14g)
Servings Per Container about 32

Amount Per Serving

Calories 90	Calories from Fat 90

	% Daily Value*
Total Fat 10g	**15%**
Saturated Fat 2g	**9%**
Polyunsaturated Fat 3g	
Monounsaturated Fat 2g	
Cholesterol 0mg	**0%**
Sodium 105mg	**4%**
Total Carbohydrate 0g	**0%**
Protein 0g	

Vitamin A 10% (25% as Beta Carotene)
Not a significant source of Dietary Fiber, Sugars, Vitamin C, Calcium and Iron
*Percent Daily Values (DV) are based on a 2,000 calorie diet.

ICE CREAM

Nutrition Facts
Serving Size 1 Tbsp (14g)
Servings Per Container about 32

Amount Per Serving

Calories 100	Calories from Fat 100

	% Daily Value*
Total Fat 11g	**17%**
Saturated Fat 7g	**36%**
Cholesterol 30mg	**10%**
Sodium 90mg	**4%**
Total Carbohydrate 0g	**0%**
Protein 0g	

Vitamin A 8%
*Percent Daily Values (DV) are based on a 2,000 calorie diet.

Look at the following comparisons. We have been taught to look at the Nutrition Facts panel—that is, the amount of carbohydrates, protein, or sugar grams—and to completely ignore whether there is any "real food" in something or not, or to check out the number of synthetic chemicals that are in a product. If any product has more than three chemicals that you cannot pronounce and doesn't look or sound like food, then it is *not* food and you don't need to eat it.

Red Baron Western Scrambler Breakfast Singles

Ingredients: Toppings: Nonfat milk, cooked pizza topping (sausage [pork, water, salt, spices, sugar], water, textured vegetable protein product [soy flour, zinc oxide, ferrous sulfate, niacinamide, calcium pantothenate, pyridoxine hydrochloride, riboflavin, thiamine mononitrate, vitamin A palmitate, vitamin B12]), cooked bacon bits, smoke flavoring added (cured with water, salt, sugar, smoke flavoring, sodium phosphates, sodium erythorbate, sodium nitrate), cheddar cheese (cultured pasteurized milk, salt, enzymes, annatto [vegetable color]), low moisture part-skim mozzarella cheese (cultured pasteurized part-skim milk, salt, enzymes), scrambled egg mix (whole eggs, skim milk, soybean oil, modified food starch, salt, xanthan gum, liquid pepper extract, citric acid, natural and artificial butter flavor, [clarified butter oil, lipolyzed butter oil, artificial flavor, annatto (color)]) green and red peppers, modified food starch, onions, dehydrated sweet cream (sweet cream, nonfat milk, lecithin), tomatoes (water, tomato paste), butter powder (butter, non-fat milk solids, sodium caseinate, BHT added to improve stability), salt, spices, smoke flavor; **Crust:** enriched flour (wheat flour, malted barley flour, niacin, iron, thiamine, riboflavin, folic acid), water, whole wheat flour, vegetable shortening (partially hydrogenated soybean oil with natural flavor and beta carotene), yeast, contains 2 percent or less of soybean oil, sugar, salt, vegetable shortening (partially hydrogenated soybean and cottonseed oils, mono and diglycerides), baking powder, dough conditioner (wheat starch, L-cysteine hydrochloride, ammonium sulfate), ascorbic acid.

Cascadian Farm Organic Indian Vegetarian Meal

Ingredients: Organic basmati rice, organic lentils, organic garbanzo beans, organic tomatoes, organic peas, organic onions, spices, organic high-oleic safflower and/or sunflower oil, organic coconut, organic sugar, sea salt, turmeric (for color).

Spend an hour or so in a good health food store, looking through the products and deciding what you like to eat and need to be eating on your particular food plan. You do not need a particular list of foods for me to give you. But here are some examples of what to eat and what not to. (The differences between the products should be obvious...)

I conducted a survey in my classes one day. I polled over a hundred and fifty people, showing them two different products and asking them which product they should eat: frozen yogurt or regular ice cream. All but one looked at the fact panel and said the yogurt. After the lecture for the day everyone understood that actually the ice cream was the real food and that after eating one scoop on a special occasion they would at least be getting some actual food and their body might even be satisfied.

I think the point is illustrated well on this example. America, we are literally poisoning ourselves!! Do *not* eat things like this!! If you had to be provided with the ingredients list

Blue Bunny Fat-Free Frozen Yogurt, Cookies & Cream

Ingredients: Pasteurized and cultured fat free milk, fat free milk solids, sugar, cookies (unbleached wheat flour, sugar, soybean oil, cocoa processed with alkali, natural caramel color, chocolate liquor, baking soda, salt, natural flavors), corn syrup, high fructose corn syrup, microcrystalline cellulose, vanilla extract, carob bean gum, guar gum, cellulose gum, carrageenan, mono & diglycerides, annatto (for color).

Breyers Natural Strawberry

Ingredients: Milk, strawberries, sugar, cream.

Parkay 70% Vegetable Oil Spread

Ingredients: Liquid soybean oil, partially hydrogenated soybean oil, whey, water, salt, vegetable mono- and diglycerides and soy lecithin (emulsifiers), sodium benzoate (to preserve freshness), artificial flavor, phosphoric acid (acidulant), vitamin A palmitate, colored with beta carotene (source of vitamin A).

Harris Teeter Salted Butter

Ingredients: Cream, Salt.

of most fast-food/junk-food "places" (I refuse to call them restaurants), you would probably never be able to eat there again. As your body heals and clears away toxins, you'll find yourself less and less able to tolerate even the smell, much less that kind of poison entering your body.

We've looked at ice cream versus yogurt, and the frozen dinners, now let's compare another common food: butter versus margarine. People often make the wrong choice when it comes to these everyday staples.

Do you see how the products shown at the top are loaded with chemicals? How the identifiable ingredients that make sense to us, like flour, cream, oil, or rice are swallowed up in a dozen other ingredients we can't even identify unless we're scientists? The real food is buried under or combined with chemicals and made toxic.

Every time I point this out to clients, they always make the same comment—"I thought I was doing so good. I was trying so hard." I know you are, but this is one of the things that is sabotaging your weight loss and preventing you from gaining your vibrant health. You'll notice on the Parkay ingredients label the manufacturer is starting to get a little tricky. Diglycerides and soy lecithin (emulsifiers), sodium benzoate (to preserve freshness)....I really don't care why they are in there; I do not want them in my body or yours. Our bodies have enough toxic chemicals to deal without us intentionally putting these kinds of things in them.

Processed food is a barrier between you and your fat-to-lean goals. Its chemical content bombards you with the very immune-stressing toxins you're working hard to eliminate. It delivers next to zero nutrients (including enzymes and fiber) but instead caters to the kind of food cravings you want to put behind you. Examine the ingredients list of any packaged, precooked, "convenient," snack or imitation food you're thinking of buying—from potato chips to frozen dinners—and let the shocking information harden your resolve to shun processed foods.

REFINED GRAINS

"Refined" is a too nice a word for a process that essentially kills everything valuable there is in wheat, rice, and other cereals and grains. It refers to a kind of milling process whereby the wheat or rice is turned white by stripping away the nutrient-containing parts and bleaching (yes, with real bleach) what remains. Often the resulting white bread or white rice is then "fortified" or "enriched" to at least pretend there's something of nutritional value in there. But, of course, the "fortification" is mostly synthetic vitamins, which add much in the way of toxic chemicals and nothing that qualifies as nutrition. Many cereals are manufactured as much as six months *before* they even get to the grocery store shelves. And many are nothing but sugar. The average appears to be between 35 and 47 percent sugar.

Eating white rice or white bread (or any pasta from refined wheat) is the equivalent of eating sugar, as far as your metabolism is concerned. Forget everything you've heard about "energy food." Refined grains convert quickly to blood sugar. Unless you're planning on running a marathon after your pancakes (another version of refined wheat flour), those pancakes are going to end up stored as fat.

There's another reason to avoid refined grains that' just as important. Like most processed foods, they offer zilch in the way of fiber. This is doubly aggravating because grains—real, whole, unrefined grains—are superb sources of fiber. Fiber, as you know, moves waste material through your intestines, discouraging constipation and toxic buildup. America is constipated today because America prefers refined grains and processed food. You can do better.

Sugar and Sugar Substitutes

The usual criticism of sugar is that it's full of "empty calories." And it's often pointed out that sugar-loaded foods like chocolate and cake are usually also packed with saturated fats. Both those observations are certainly true, but I'm afraid the problem with sugar goes beyond that. The human body simply isn't designed to process sugar in concentrated forms like pure cane sugar, especially the bleached and refined table sugar version. Thus, sugar acts as a toxin in your body, weakening your immune system. It's associated with all kinds of disease, from diabetes and gout to heart disease and kidney problems. Just as bad, not only is sugar something that's craved, it also induces cravings. The sugar that you swallow after giving in to your doughnut craving acts more like a drug in your body than a food.

It's quickly absorbed, causing an intense reaction. Your blood sugar level soars (of course), giving you a burst of short-lived energy. But that sugar rush also forces an emergency release of insulin to balance out your blood sugar level. The resulting rapid fall in your blood sugar level triggers more sugar cravings, and the vicious cycle starts anew.

Do you see why the expression "sugar addict" is to be taken literally? Keep in mind also that the table sugar you use to sweeten food and the sugar-laden desserts you end your meals with are just part of the story. Check the ingredients list of just about any packaged and/or processed foods—even foods that aren't "sweet" in the slightest—and you'll usually find sugar in some form. Whether it's called sucrose, dextrose, glucose, fructose, maltose, or corn sweetener, it's sugar. Your nutraplenishing will help you get off the sugar roller coaster by diminishing your cravings. But it's going to take some determination on your part to overcome what may be a lifetime sugar habit and get your intake down to manageable levels. It's never easy to kick any addiction, but I know you can do it with the help of your nutrients.

Whatever you do, though, don't even consider switching to sugar substitutes. Pouring more toxins into your body will only make things worse. And make no mistake about it, that's exactly what you're doing when you swallow "diet" soft drinks laced with such artificial sweeteners as aspartame (in Equal), saccharine (in Sweet'N Low), or any other synthetic chemical. Don't let label teasers like "diet," "no calories," and "no sugar" fool you. An artificial sweetener is no friend in your fat-to-lean quest. At least sugar comes from food. The artificial sweeteners have been linked to all kinds of problems, including obesity. I would rather you drink a "regular" soft drink and wean off of them as your body heals and strengthens than ever drink one more "diet" drink.

DANGEROUS FATS

Too much dietary fat means too much body fat. But so does a misguided fear of fat. It never ceases to amaze me how much junk people will eat as long as it's labeled "low fat." Yes, if you're used to the typical American diet, you probably need to cut down on your overall dietary fat. But that doesn't mean that anything that's low in fat is a healthy food. And it certainly doesn't mean that you should never eat any fat. On the contrary, a moderate amount of fat is absolutely necessary for a balanced diet, for satisfying meals, and for weight loss.

What's more, certain kinds of fat are health promoting; you most likely need to be consuming more of them, not less. You want to reduce your overall fat consumption by cutting out the bad fats in favor of the good ones.

Since we're going over problem foods right now, let's take a simple look at the fats to avoid. You do need to cut down as much as possible on fat from animal food. This is mostly saturated fat, which has long been known to raise your levels of the dangerous form of cholesterol. That doesn't require eliminating all animal foods from your diet—in fact, I don't recommend doing that.

But you do want to choose the leanest cuts of red meat (hormone-free, of course). You want to remove the skin from chicken and turkey. And you want to learn to choose something else besides heavy cheeses and fatty meats like bacon.

What's most important, however, is that you completely eliminate oils that have been artificially altered. For the most part, that means cutting out what's known as hydrogenated oils or trans fats. These are oils that have been tampered with chemically. They're what make margarine firm like butter. They're also found in a wide array of processed foods like mayonnaise, pancake mix, cereals, candies, frozen foods, and salad dressings. They're virtually unavoidable in commercially baked products like cookies, pies, cakes, and crackers.

Again, by avoiding processed foods, you've done most of the work needed to eliminate hydrogenated oils from your diet. The federal government has recently recognized the cholesterol-raising dangers of hydrogenated oils and imposed new labeling requirements, making it easier for you to spot this unnatural fat and steer clear of anything that contains it.

DAIRY PRODUCTS

Most of my clients come to me eating too much dairy. I'm not advocating cutting out all dairy food. I'm definitely not suggesting that you switch to "dairy substitutes." Artificial food is never a better choice. I'd much rather you eat real eggs every day than one Egg-Beater.

What I do suggest, however, is that you reduce or eliminate your consumption of at least two milk products—cheese and milk itself. Some yogurts are ok—there are organic brands that contain no added sugar. You can add some real fruit to it. If you notice that your allergies act up or your sinuses get inflamed after eating this, then stay away from it.

I've already mentioned the heavy load of saturated fat in cheese. Cheese can also increase fungus or candida in your system. Yeast and/or candida problems are a very large road block to weight loss and health building. So just do not eat cheese. The problem gets worse when you melt the cheese or use it in cooking, since you're now eating heat-damaged as well as saturated fat. Grown-ups who care about their health don't eat nachos and pizza.

And milk? American milk isn't sterilized, as it is in many European countries. That's why we have to refrigerate it and they don't. Milk introduces toxic bacteria into your system, and can result in inflammation from your body's efforts to get rid of them. Most milk on the market passes along the toxins imposed upon the cows—the pesticides and herbicides in the food they eat, and the antibiotics and hormones injected into them. Whole milk is high in saturated fat, and the so-called 2 percent milk isn't all that much lower. Many people are allergic to milk; others are lactose intolerant.

Milk just isn't worth it. But what about the calcium it provides? What will replace it? A combination of things. Fregetables deliver the calcium that such vegetables as kale, collard greens, broccoli, spinach, and parsley would provide if they weren't nutrient depleted. Sardines, salmon, and shrimp are also rich in calcium. And because you're working toward re-ducing or eliminating such things as saturated fat, salt, sugar, and caf-feinated beverages, you'll utilize the calcium you do get much more efficiently. If you or your doctor still feel it's necessary, supplements are available that provide calcium from natural sources that your body can ab-sorb (as opposed to calcium carbonate).

SOFT DRINKS

The only thing I can think of that's worse for your health and weight-loss goals than soft drinks are diet soft drinks. They're loaded with sugar or sugar substitutes like aspartame. Most have caffeine, which you must avoid except for the controlled amounts in your Masters of Metabolism nutri-ents. Less known but even more devastating is the calcium-depleting ef-fect of the phosphates that are in all soft drinks, diet or otherwise. Nothing leaches calcium out of your bones more than soft drinks do. You can take all the calcium substitutes you can get your hands on, but if you're drinking colas every day, you've got a date with osteoporosis.

There are no ifs, ands, or buts about soft drinks. If you care about get-ting lean and reclaiming your vibrant health, please, please, please drink something else besides these vile concoctions. Make up your mind, find some alternatives, and increase your water intake. Don't try to do it all at once, but make the effort—if you want to lose weight and gain your vi-brant health, that is. If you have been on your nutrients for more than a month, this should not be as difficult as if you haven't started them yet. My client Sam was addicted to diet cokes for over fifteen years. Within two weeks on the nutrients, not only had he lost 10 pounds, but he called to tell me he couldn't believe it—not only was he off diet soft drinks but he couldn't even stand the thought of one.

FERMENTED FOODS

Pickled foods, vinegary foods, and alcohol drinks are the fermented foods you should limit. This is especially important if you're what I call a "yeast baby"—that is, prone to bloating and infections from an overabundance of yeast in your system. Reason? Fermented foods have microscopic mold in them, which is toxic to your body. This holds true for alcohol too. In fact, think about what the term "intoxicated" really means. It's what happens when your liver can't handle the overload of a substance that doesn't belong in your body (that is, a toxin—in this case, the alcohol). A hangover is simply the effects you feel of your body still trying to deal with the toxicity. Would an occasional glass or two of wine derail your fat-to-lean express? Probably not. But I look at it this way: I just spent the last four years of my life detoxing my system. So I'm always going to think twice before intentionally introducing more toxins. I'm not perfect, but I know the price and I usually don't want to pay it.

SALT

Our food is so oversalted that even if it were totally benign I'd still recommend reducing it in your diet! The truth is, though, that excess salt plays a role in the development of high blood pressure, especially among those who are salt-sensitive. Too much salt has also been connected with fluid retention, premenstrual syndrome, headaches, and constipation. One way or another, all that salt is keeping your VHI lower than it should be.

It may surprise you to learn that only about a quarter of your salt intake comes out of the salt shaker in your kitchen or on your table. Most of the salt you eat is already included in packaged, canned, and processed foods. This is yet another example of how eliminating processed foods from your diet automatically takes care of most of your other food concerns.

Another thing you may not have known is that the kind of salt generally found in markets has plenty of detrimental effects. Typical table salt (and the salt in processed foods) is "mined," heat processed, and highly refined so that it consists of nothing but sodium chloride. Some sea salt, on the other hand, contains as many as eighty-two trace minerals. It's that balance that is thought to account for sea salt's healthier reputation.

SO NOW WHAT?

As you read through that "little shopping list of horrors," a few thoughts may have run through your mind.

"I eat every one of those foods all the time!" So do most people. You are by no means alone. In reality, you should be very encouraged that your course is so clear. Unlike most people, you have clearly identified the habits you need to adjust to turn your health around and start shedding that unwelcome fat.

"This is an overwhelming list. How can I possibly cut out all those foods?" Don't try. Not all at once, anyway. And not yet. First of all, every component of the Nashville Diet is to be phased in slowly and comfortably. You start nutraplenishing slowly. You ease into your detox regimen. You start off with just a little bit of exercise. And you will gradually start cutting down on the problem foods you may be used to — one at a time.

Also, don't let the scope of the "problem" list overwhelm you. Think of what you've just read as information only. You are not under orders to eliminate all those foods immediately, and for good reason. It makes no sense to concentrate on what not to eat before you know what you should be eating. And that's the good news. For every toxin-drenched, nutrient-challenged, harmful food on the list above, there are healthy, satisfying, and delicious alternatives. Those are what we'll look at in the next chapter. Some of the alternatives are old friends you'll recognize. Others will be new experiences. All of them will move you closer to vibrant health. And all of them will speed you on your journey from fat to lean.

THE SOLUTION:

real food for real people

at some point in their recovery, a question occurs to many of my clients that may have occurred to you. Why, they want to know, do we have to eat at all? Don't the nutraceuticals we're taking deliver the nutrients we need in food form? Wouldn't we lose weight faster if we just stopped eating and took the nutrients? The answer to that last question is, well, yes. However, the weight you'd be losing would be more muscle than fat. The short-term outcome would be illness accompanied by muscle wasting and pain. And if you keep it up long enough, you'll be dead. But, yes, you'll lose weight. Is that what you want? Of course not.

Not long ago I had a general physical. I went to my old family doctor who had treated me during much of my illness. The last time I'd seen him he had been quite overweight and noticeably exhausted. Now, three years later, I was stunned at how thin and emaciated he looked. He was so gaunt and sickly I was afraid at first that he had cancer or AIDS.

When he left the room, I asked the nurse if there was something wrong with him. No, she said, he had simply lost weight—as though it were a good thing. When I saw him again, I had to ask how he'd lost so much weight. The answer didn't surprise me. "I just stopped eating," he told me. If you need living proof that intense calorie deprivation is a misguided and unhealthy approach to weight loss, look no further than that doctor.

My friends, you *have* to eat. In the next chapter, we'll see why (contrary to my doctor's approach) you have to eat in order to lose fat. Right now, though, I'll give you three answers to the question of why we nutraplenished wonders have to eat at all.

- ☐ Food provides the raw material in the form of building blocks that gives your body what it needs to build rather than break down.
- ☐ Food, not your nutrients, provides the energy (calories) to run your metabolic engine.
- ☐ Food, not your nutrients, provides fiber that our bodies need to function properly.

While the nutrients provide what today's food supply is missing—the "micronutrients" to nourish your cells—food supplies what the nutrients can't. If you like, you can think of food as supplementing your nutrient intake. How's that for an ironic twist?

Since food is necessary, the challenge is to eat food that will provide the raw material, fiber, and energy without jeopardizing health, raising toxicity levels, or increasing body fat. We've already learned that there are plenty of foods that do as much harm as good. Unfortunately, those are precisely the foods that are most widely available and therefore eaten in our society. Now it's time to learn about the foods that deliver what we need without the harmful side effects. Fortunately, there are plenty of those as well. Your mission is to make the transition from problem foods to healthy foods. So let's get going!

SEVEN SIMPLE GUIDELINES FOR FAT-TO-LEAN EATING

I encourage you to learn as much as you can about the science of nutrition and how your body processes food. At the same time, though, I don't think you need a degree in food sciences to start eating the kinds of foods that will help you maintain a healthy weight as you improve your overall health. Yet most diet books seem to be competing with each other to see which can pack in the most detailed nutritional science. That's fine, except for one thing. You're probably long overdue for a change in eating habits. And once your nutraplenishing has balanced your system and reduced your cravings enough to make such a change feasible, there's no reason to wade through an advanced course in nutrition before you get started.

That's especially true when you realize that the changes themselves are really quite simple. What you need to do can be summarized in seven basic guidelines.

The guidelines are specific enough to ensure that you'll be eating in a way that promotes fat loss. But they are by no means a strictly regimented food program. There are enough good foods in this world to allow you unlimited choices within the guidelines. The Nashville Diet doesn't feed you; it teaches you to feed yourself in healthy, lean-promoting ways.

If you keep taking your nutrients, eat without cravings, and follow these simple guidelines, you will turn your eating habits around and overcome another barrier between you and vibrant health.

1. Eat "Live" Food, Not Processed Food

If you do nothing else but faithfully follow this one vital eating guideline, you'll have done more for your vibrant health than a thousand fad diets could ever offer. What's more, incorporating the "live food" idea almost automatically takes care of most of the other food guidelines I'm recommending.

But I must tell you, emphasizing live food over processed food is no minor adjustment if you're used to the typical American way of eating. It's a big change, but a doable one, especially if you've been taking your nutrients.

What do I mean by live food? Simply put, it's food that comes to you as nature intended. It's real food that hasn't been altered much from the way it came out of the ground or water, or off the tree or land. It's pure food without additives, chemicals, preservatives, "enrichment," or any kind of processing.

Does that sound restrictive? Hardly! Live food as a category offers you most of the menu that sustained humankind for eons up until the second half of the twentieth century, when it started getting pushed aside in favor of processed food, fast food, and junk food—and the resulting obesity.

Live food includes all fresh fruits and vegetables, legumes, nuts, beans, seeds, whole grains, clean meat and fish, eggs, and more. If you put a roast in the oven and serve it with peas, brown rice, mushrooms sautéed in olive oil, and a salad of greens and tomato with a dressing made from olive oil and garden herbs, you've prepared an entirely live meal.

But if you unpack and heat up the "convenient" alternative to the same meal, you'll probably eliminate everything "live" about it. You'll be eating a laboratory full of chemicals, empty refined white rice, hydrogenated oils, etc.

Live food doesn't mean that nothing you eat can come from a bag or a package or jar. Vine-ripened is best, of course, but frozen fruits and vegetables qualify as live food. That bag of frozen peas is a fine choice, as long as that bag's full of very cold peas only, and not a lot of chemicals or salt or butter flavoring.

Finding the live food in packages or jars requires some label inspection on your part. For example, fresh, raw unsalted peanuts are clearly a live food. But so are dry-roasted, unsalted peanuts. Taking it a step farther, peanut butter in the jar is fine, too—as long as the ingredients list includes nothing but peanuts. The sugared-up, chemically laden processed peanut butter that usually goes on kids' sandwiches (on heavily refined white bread, of course) has no place in your fat-to-lean plans. So read that label!

2. FEAST ON FRESH FRUITS AND VEGETABLES

Why am I telling you to eat a lot of fruits and vegetables after going on so much about how nutrient-depleted they are? Because fruits and vegetables deliver bulk and fiber and energy without saturated fat. Because they help prevent constipation. Because they regulate blood sugar. And because they provide a healthy live food to satisfy your hunger without resorting to problem foods. Since you have to eat, eat fruits and vegetables.

By the way, don't be confused by some "expert" diet advice that cautions against certain fruits or vegetables because of their natural sugar content or incompatibility with complicated diet objectives. This is the kind of overdetailed diet instruction that turns people off from eating healthy. Fruits and vegetables are great live foods! As long as you're not sprinkling sugar or pouring cream over it, eat any fruit you want. (At some point, when you have learned and implemented the basics of the Nashville Diet, you may need to limit some fruit intake for certain body imbalances.) And as long as you keep it away from butter or margarine or mayonnaise or creamy dressings or rich sauces or vinegary liquid or any other non–live companion, eat any fresh vegetable you want. But in the meantime, please choose live food!

3. Choose Whole Grains and Cereals

Eliminating processed grains and cereals and avoiding refined flour is a lot easier to do when you're aware of all the wonderful alternatives out there. First and foremost, make sure any bread or cereal you choose is made from whole grain—that is, wheat (or whatever other grain) that hasn't had its fiber-rich parts milled out of it. Not only do whole grains provide the fiber you need for good digestion and regular bowel movements, they also tend to convert to blood sugar more slowly, which is a definite metabolic plus for your fat-to-lean goal. It's simple to discern if a bread or cereal is made from whole grain—it will say so right on the label. Don't be fooled by ambiguous terms like "healthy" or "natural." They tell you nothing. Also, though white bread is now a thing of the past for you, a brownish bread color doesn't necessarily indicate whole grain. And remember that "multigrain" simply means more than one kind of grain. Whether it's made from whole grain or not is another matter. Check the ingredients list.

Your rice and pasta must also be whole grain. That basically implies switching from white rice to brown rice. Whole-wheat pasta is not what you usually see, but it's out there. If you must eat pasta, find the whole-grain version and stick to it.

Needless to say, the whole-grain factor isn't the only issue with your cereals. You want to search the shelves for products that aren't loaded up with sugar, synthetic "vitamins," preservatives, and other chemicals. Again, ignore buzz words like "natural" and "healthy," which can mean whatever the manufacturers want them to mean. And don't be taken in by those Eden-like garden scenes that seem to be on every package of commercial cereal these days—that's marketing, not information.

Again, check the ingredients list. Also, explore the bulk bins at health food stores for the best whole-grain choices. One more thing: Expand your grain horizons beyond whole wheat and whole grain rice. Variety is always helpful when you're trying to balance your system (which you are!), and there are some incredible grains available that most folks have never even seen, let alone tried. Here are five I particularly recommend:

Quinoa. It's pronounced KEEN-wa and it goes great with any meal. It cooks like rice (1 cup quinoa to 2 cups water), so it's a fine alternative to brown rice or couscous. It has 50 percent more protein than wheat, as well as more iron, more calcium, more phosphorus, and more natural vitamins A, E, and B.

As a gluten-free, whole-grain flour, quinoa was a staple of the Incas. Today it makes wonderful breads and biscuits if you combine one part of it with four parts whole-wheat flour.

Spelt. With its delicious light, nutty flavor, spelt is a good choice for getting off refined flour if you don't care for the taste of whole wheat. You can readily substitute spelt flour for wheat in baking recipes as long as you reduce the liquid by 25 percent. It also works great as a pilaf-like dish. Presoak it for eighty minutes (1 cup spelt to 3 cups water) and then bring it to a boil in the same water. Simmer it covered for an hour or ninety minutes.

Amaranth. It was the grain of the Aztecs—gluten free and slightly spicy with a sticky, gelatinous texture. For a side dish, cook 1 cup of amaranth to 3 cups water. You can also pop it like popcorn. The flour form of amaranth is also gluten free. Use it as an "accent" flour; its flavor is too strong to use alone to make waffles, cookies, or muffins. Don't use it in recipes that require baking yeast.

Steel-cut oats. Steel-cut oats are whole grain oats that have been steamed and coarsely cut with steel blades, reducing the cooking time from ninety to thirty minutes. All the cholesterol-lowering oat bran is there. As a hot breakfast cereal, its taste and texture are slightly different from traditional oatmeal. Just bring 3 cups of water to a boil, add 1 cup of the steel-cut oats, cover, and simmer for thirty minutes over low heat. They also make a great addition to long-cooking soups.

Barley. Whole barley is rich in protein, potassium, and calcium. It's great as a breakfast porridge, since it expands with water to four times its dry size. Cook 1 cup of barley to 3 cups of water, simmering for twenty minutes after bringing it to a quick boil.

Barley is chewy, so you can actually make tasty barley burgers. Mix 2 cups of cooked barley with 1 cup shredded vegetables, some onion and garlic, and an egg. Form the mixture into patties and bake.

4. STICK TO THE GOOD FATS

I've asked you to limit fats in your diet. I've also asked you to eliminate saturated fat as much as possible. Saturated fats are primarily of animal origin and solidify at room temperature. You're getting saturated fat when you eat any of the following foods: beef, pork, lamb, cold cuts, sausage, bacon, hot dogs, cheeses, butter, ice cream, sour cream, whole milk, eggs, turkey skin, chicken skin, and many processed foods.

I've also asked you to eliminate all fat in the form of hydrogenated oils, also known as trans fats. That you can accomplish by replacing processed foods with live food, and avoiding margarine, mayonnaise, and most packaged baked goods. But I am not asking you to strive to eliminate *all* fat from your diet. That would be counterproductive. Remember the golden rule of the Nashville Diet: Your body seeks balance. If you deny it any dietary fat at all, it will consider itself "fat starved" and will hold on tight to its own body fat. In other words, you must eat some (dietary) fat to lose (body) fat. Like an oil change for our car. Old toxic cellulite-ridden "oil" out and good clean new "oil" in. Our body is "sealed" like a vacuum and will not "let something go" until it is properly replaced.

The trick is to replace the bad fats (saturated, hydrogenated, and many oils) with a limited amount of good fats, which fall under the category of unsaturated (either mono- or polyunsaturated). Entire books have been written on healthy fat choices, but, as always, we're going to keep it simple here. The following are the good fats you want to choose:

"Oily" fish. Here I'm talking about salmon, mackerel, sardines, herring, eel, rainbow trout, and the like. Aside from the protein they deliver, these are superb sources for the most important kind of polyunsaturated fat for your body—omega-3 fatty acids.

Nuts and seeds. These deliver omega-6 and omega-3 fatty acids, the two most important kinds of beneficial unsaturated (in this case, polyunsaturated) fats.

Flax oil. Take this like a supplement, a teaspoonful every day. Flaxseed is by far the richest source of alpha-linolenic acid, the key omega-3. Get it from the refrigerated section of your health food store.

Olive oil. Here's a monounsaturated fat that helps digestion; fights the harmful LDL type of cholesterol; slows down the aging of skin, bones, and joints; and is even said to protect against certain forms of cancer. It's more suited for human consumption than any other oil, and is more easily tolerated by the stomach.

Olive oil will be one of your best friends as you follow the Nashville Diet eating guidelines. It's what you'll put on salads instead of the creamy or processed dressings that you've bid adieu to. It's what you'll dip your (whole-grain) bread in instead of slathering it with butter or margarine. And, of course, you can cook with it instead of margarine, butter, lard, or any of the harmful oils. Look for cold-pressed, extra-virgin olive oil, which is the least processed. And you'll want it in an opaque (not clear) container.

Sesame oil. As long as it's unrefined, sesame oil is the best to cook with. Sesame oil has almost equal amounts of polyunsaturated and mononounsaturated fat, and stays stable at high temperatures better than other oils. While occasional sautéing or stir-frying with sesame or olive oil is fine and tasty, avoid fried food in general. Frying with animal fat will expose you to too much bad (saturated) fat, while unsaturated oils (especially polyunsaturated oils) tend to be damaged by the high temperature, thus turning into as harmful a product as hydrogenated oil.

Are there other suitable fat sources? Yes there are, and I invite you to investigate this fascinating nutritional topic more thoroughly on your own. For our purposes now, however, stick to the above five fat recommendations, and keep the amounts low. If you consciously choose no other fat but those, your ratio of good fat to bad fat will be light years better than almost everybody else's.

5. Choose Lean Meats for Protein

You need to eat meat because you need the protein. Protein is the raw material you build your body with, including the muscle mass that's so vital to your fat-to-lean plans. Your nutrients deliver some important amino acids (the building blocks of protein), but they cannot replace meat as a protein source. I eat meat regularly, and I think you should too. I know that advice contradicts the leanings of many in the field of "natural" or "alternative" nutrition, who tend to lean toward a vegetarian lifestyle. Can you get all the amino acids you need on a vegetarian diet? It's possible, but I don't think very many people manage to do it. A vegetarian is just as likely to be sick or overweight as a meat eater, and probably more likely to be muscle wasted. (Once you have the basics of the Nashville Diet down, some body imbalances might require that you eat an almost vegetarian diet for a short period to lose fat. Once you are where you want your body to be, size-wise, then you'll need to start eating meat again.)

So don't feel you need to eliminate meat from your diet to be healthy. Concentrate instead on eliminating the processed foods. Eat meat three or four days a week, and fish the other three or four. To minimize the saturated fat, choose lean cuts of red meat (filet is best) or skinless white meat (chicken or turkey). Keep the portion reasonable—as you work your way toward fat burning and meal size reductions, a good rule of thumb is the volume of two of your own fists. Avoid ground meat, cured meat, or fat-marbled cuts like prime rib. Especially avoid any kind of processed meat, such as sausage, bacon, frankfurters, or cold cuts.

6. EAT ORGANIC

All of the first five food guidelines raise issues of toxicity. You can deal with that problem by going out of your way to buy only organic food. This is not nearly as difficult to do as it once was, but it's still going to be a challenge if you're not used to it. It's true that some supermarkets are carrying more and more organic products, but you'll find fresher produce at your health food store and farmer's markets. It's worth the time and effort.

The United States Department of Agriculture (USDA) now has labeling rules for organic products. Foods labeled "100 percent organic" must contain only organically produced raw or processed products. For those labeled simply "organic," the required amount is 95 percent. Any food or food product with more than 5 percent nonorganic ingredients cannot be labeled organic.

Remember, organic produce is not necessarily more nutrient-rich than the rest, since it can be subject to the same soil-depletion and green-harvesting problems. Nor is it always going to be completely free of any chemical residue, since wandering chemicals know no boundaries. But at least you know that it was grown and harvested free of synthetic fertilizers, pesticides, herbicides, and other poisons. Whatever extra you pay for organic is very much worth it. Remember that the organic advantage is by no means limited to fresh fruits and vegetables. You can find certified organic versions of just about any food you might put on your table, including frozen dinners.

What are you getting when you buy organic? You're getting food that was grown and processed with no genetic modification, no hormones (important for your meat!), no antibiotics (important for your meat and poultry!), no pesticides, no herbicides, no insecticides, and no irradiation. The absence of all of those unwelcome extras is essential for the detox component of your fat-to-lean strategy. Organic is no longer a word for the fringe element. It is vital for your vibrant health.

7. NEVER SET FOOT IN A FAST-FOOD RESTAURANT AGAIN

You know the ones I'm talking about. There's no surer way to break every one of the previous six guidelines than to order something at any of the chain-style junk food joints that have over-run our country and the world. It's not just the flood of saturated fats and cholesterol and refined flour that they're famous for. The food is also loaded with higher-than-average amounts of pesticides and other chemicals.

I'm always shocked when I see so-called experts who supposedly are trying to help people get healthy include in their diet books ways to "eat responsibly" at fast-food places. But honestly, you can't do it. Unless you really don't want your body and health back. All you're going to get is processed and refined, nutrient-depleted, pesticide-riddled food-like substances made with bad oils and the wrong meats, served in outrageously oversized portions.

As you can tell, I feel rather strongly about this subject. I've seen too many toxic and overweight clients who've nearly lost all hope after a lifetime of eating habits shaped by the fast-food mentality. The truth is, there's no reason for you to even look at one of these places again, let alone walk into one. If you do, throw this book away first, and tell yourself honestly, "I'd rather eat here than have my vibrant health." There is no compromise—it's one or the other.

SMART CHOICES FOR SMART EATERS

In this chapter I've tried to concentrate on promoting the good food that's available to you instead of warning you again about the unhealthy problem foods. Still, most of my clients tend to feel a little discouraged, if not outright annoyed, about the prospect of no longer eating some foods that they've always enjoyed. I imagine you might feel the same.

The best way to get through the transition is to explore the infinite possibilities contained in the realm of healthy food that I've described in the guidelines I've just given you. One thing that helps is to sort of "prime the pump" of your imagination by offering some specific alternatives to some specific problem foods.

Here are some of my favorite switches. There are of course, countless others for you to discover.

Instead of sugar...

try a naturally sweet herb called stevia, available in most health food stores. It doesn't work well for cooking recipes, but it's a wonderful sweetener for iced tea and most other drinks, and for hot cereal.

Instead of sugar for cooking...

use fructose. It's also a sugar, but it's from fruit rather than cane or beets. It doesn't race your insulin and shoot your blood sugar up and down rapidly.

Instead of refined cane sugar...

go for organic raw pure cane sugar. Again, it's still sugar and should be limited, but because the white sugar hasn't been mechanically separated, it won't have as much of the drug-like effect as the superconcentrated white sugar, and it actually has some minerals left in it.

Instead of candy...

enjoy grapes for a sweet treat. As you overcome the addiction-like sugar habit, the natural sweetness of grapes will seem wonderful. Keep some in the freezer for a dessert-like interlude.

Instead of sodas...

drink sparkling waters. Fruit-flavored versions with raspberry or lemon-lime (among others) help keep ex-soda junkies on the soft-drink wagon. Make sure there's no sugar added.

Instead of sodas...

drink iced herb teas. Whatever herb tea (as opposed to caffeinated black or green tea) you like will be just as good served cold. Fruity herb teas of raspberry, blueberry, or blackberry are delicious over ice. I'm talking about actual herb tea, not what is normally served in restaurants of regular caffeinated tea with canned, sugared orange and pineapple juice added. You can get many real herbal teas in tea bags, steep them in boiling water, add stevia for sweetness, then chill. You can also carry these herbal tea bags along with you and ask for hot water, for a yummy hot drink.

Instead of salt...

try one of the many herb blends on the market to spice up any dish. Your taste for salt was just a habit. Why not switch it for a less harmful and equally tasty habit? There are so many blends (or individual spices) available that you're sure to find one you'll want to use often. Broaden your taste horizons! Experiment! Make your trips to the health food store an adventure. (It's really easy to get kids into something like this as you teach them how to have their own vibrant health for a lifetime. You don't want them to fight the same health and weight issues you are, so train them now. Start with a fun, new, tasty, healthy "salt.")

Instead of salt...

use fresh onions and garlic as you cook.

Instead of crackers and chips...

dry-roast some unsalted raw nuts and nibble judiciously. You're substituting good oils for bad oils, and live food for processed food. I like to put pecans, walnuts, and almonds on a flat cookie sheet, sprinkle a little herb seasoning over them and perhaps a few drops of olive oil, and bake them at 375 degrees for about twenty minutes, turning them over about every five minutes. They end up crunchier and more delicious than any chip or cracker could hope to be.

Instead of milk...

use milk made from oats (which of course isn't really milk at all). You'll find it next to the soy milk in the natural food section, but I recommend it over soy milk, which is harder on the kidneys. Oat milk is naturally sweet and creamy, perfect for smoothies or for pouring over cold cereal.

Instead of canned tuna...

eat canned salmon. Both offer protein and healthy omega-3 oils, but the salmon is less likely to deliver mercury toxicity. Salmon's also not as associated with mayonnaise and white bread, both of which you've left behind along the road from fat to lean. I've found canned salmon to be really good with an herbal mustard on pecan or almond nut crackers.

A CHANGE OF HABIT

There are two unwavering truths about the healthy-eating aspect of the Nashville Diet. One is that everything you need to know about what to eat is contained in the seven simple food guidelines we've just gone over.

The other truth is that no matter how simple these guidelines are, longtime habits take time to change. You know and I know that it's just as easy and satisfying to use olive oil as margarine, but actually implementing that knowledge is another matter. Old tendencies have a momentum of their own that takes effort to slow down and turn around. But they can be overcome!

Believe me, I can sympathize. I was at one time a chocoholic to the nth degree. Even when I started to come around to healthy eating and re-gaining my vibrant health, I never imagined that I'd stop indulging my chocolate-tooth. But it turns out that I had overcome my addiction without even being aware of it. I know this because a neighbor of mine one day mentioned that she'd noticed I no longer ate chocolate. We were the kind of friends who could wander in and out of each other's houses without formalities, and she had always left brownies for me on her kitchen counter. "You haven't touched one of my brownies in weeks," she told me. And she was right. I'd completely forgotten about those brownies. But here's the kicker. Just to see what would happen, I took a bite of one. And you know what? I nearly spit it out; it was disgusting to me. I haven't eaten chocolate since, and don't have the least desire to.

So old habits *can* be overcome. As long as you truly want to do it, you'll eventually trade in all those bad eating habits for the good ones embodied in our seven guidelines — and you'll feel more satisfied, not less.

Nutraplenishing smooths the way because it reduces the crave factor that makes sensible eating so difficult. But let's face it, if you've been eating your meals out of cans and packages all your life, committing to live food is going to take some dedication and persistence. Let me share with you some strategies that have helped my clients make the transition from fat-inducing food to healthy eating.

Take it slow. The one-step-at-a-time approach you're using for every facet of the Nashville Diet, from nutraplenishing through detox work and exercise, applies with your food program as well. Don't even consider overhauling your entire diet at once. Wean yourself off the bad stuff as you slowly integrate the good stuff.

Prioritize. Make a list of four or five "bad" things you often eat or drink — soft drinks, sweets, saturated fat, or anything else we've talked about in this chapter and the previous one. Put them in order based on how hard you think it will be to give them up in favor of a healthier alternative. Then start working your way up the list, implementing the changes starting with the easiest. A realistic pace might be that you eliminate one item per week.

Get to know your local health food store. If you've never shopped in a health food store, you're in for a pleasant surprise. Gone are the days of a few bins of spotty-looking produce and a shelf or two of supplements. The selection is immense at many stores and the presentation enticing. But it's still a strange (though wonderful) new world, so the more browsing around and exploring you do, the better you'll be able to avail yourself of the possibilities.

Be an avid label reader. That's really the only way you can tell what you're buying and eating. Some of the things you want to check are the kind of fat in any food product, whether the grains (if any) are refined, if there's any added sugar, and if it's organic. If you're in a mainstream supermarket or convenience store, pay extra attention to any possible additives or chemicals. If there are names on the ingredient list that don't sound like food, don't buy the product.

It's not all or nothing. Don't expect to eat 100 percent organic food. You can't eliminate every single processed food from your diet. There's going to be some saturated fat in some of your food. Sugar's going to sneak in here and there. We don't live in a perfect world, so don't be discouraged. Just make a conscious effort to eat as much live food as possible, eliminate as much processed food as you can, and abandon completely those problem foods over which you do have control (soft drinks, for example).

Get creative. Once you learn that a meal is something you prepare rather than unpack, a world of possibilities opens up. Not only can you get creative in the way you prepare food, there are lots of new horizons to be explored in your meal selection. Our seven guidelines allow for endless food choices. Stroll the health food aisles, read some labels, and take home something within the guidelines that you've never tried before. Eating the same five or ten dishes all the time (as most Americans do) is unhealthy, not to mention boring. Explore!

Assert yourself. There's no reason you can't eat out and stay within the guidelines. Choose restaurants that are more likely to serve live food. Then don't be afraid to ascertain just what it is you're getting. It's not rude or pushy to ask if a dish is prepared with lard, or if the salmon is served with a butter sauce. Nor is it out of line to request an extra pile of vegetables instead of the white rice. It's your food and your money and your health. You have the right to ask for what you want.

from fat to lean—
the nashville way

believe it or not, you've already mastered the basic knowledge
necessary to put the Nashville Diet into action. Surprised? It's true. You've
promised yourself that you'll improve your health in order to lose weight,
not the other way around. You now know that the path from fat to lean begins with a balanced system. You've become aware that toxicity is the
hidden enemy of fat loss. And you've learned that just a few key changes
in the foods you choose are all the "diet" instruction you need.

That's it. In fact, if I'm asked to summarize the Nashville Diet requirements in twenty-five words or less, I can do it without hesitation:

*Take your nutrients to eliminate cravings. Detoxify your system. Avoid
new toxic exposure as much as possible. Exercise. Eat live food instead of
processed food.*

There you go. Twenty-five words exactly! Do those things and you'll
be leaner, healthier and happier—for the rest of your life. What could be
simpler? Oh, *drink plenty of clean water.* Extra five—not too bad.

Scientists will tell you that the most elegant and beautiful theories are
the simplest. And I'm convinced that the basic simplicity of the Nashville

Diet is a big reason why everybody who follows the Nashville Diet program is so ecstatic with their results. For one thing, it's easy to follow. More important, you'll find yourself better able to stick with it, since you're nourishing and cleaning your body rather than starving it.

Still, most of my clients are as surprised as you probably are at the basic approach of the Nashville Diet. They wonder, "Where's the sacrifice? Where's the pain? Where's the calorie chart? How come I'm not counting grams of this and percentages of that? Why am I not being told exactly what to eat at each meal? Where's the super-protein strategy? Or the carbo-loading strategy? Or the fat-free strategy? Where's the lose-twenty-pounds-in-twenty-minutes promise?"

My response to each of those questions (and a thousand others in the same vein) is the same: They reflect a mindset that has no place here. They belong to a school of dieting that never, ever works in the long run, and not all that often in the short run. The goal of those diets is to get your weight down *now*, one way or the other.

But just as a yo-yo rolls back up after you throw it down, so will your weight. There are two obvious reasons why yo-yo diets act like yo-yos. One is that they ignore the health factors that lead to food cravings and fat retention (mainly nutrient depletion and toxin accumulation). The other is that they impose unnatural eating requirements that nobody can obey for very long (especially if those requirements include some kind of calorie deprivation, which most of them do). One fad diet differs from another only in what new eating gimmick it comes up with. But the worst thing about yo-yo diets isn't just that they don't work, but that they actually make you fatter in the long run. And in so doing, they make it more difficult to turn things around when you finally decide to do things the healthy way. When all is said and done, yo-yo diets are unhealthy. So before I present two modest "diet" strategies that are compatible with the Nashville Diet approach, let's take a look at how your diet goals differ from those of the yo-yo dieters.

WHEN THE FAT HITS THE FIRE

Here's something you should always keep in mind as you follow my program: Your goal is not to lose weight. Surprised you again, haven't I? "Dr. Marilyn's gone off the deep end this time," you're probably thinking. "I sure as shootin' didn't pick up this book to *gain* weight!" Actually, you picked up this book to lose fat. Losing fat and losing weight is not the same thing. Sure, we often say "lose weight" when we mean "lose fat." I've used that euphemism myself in this book. But it's not accurate. What you weigh is not based solely on how much fat you're burdened with, but also on what's called your lean body mass, which includes muscle mass. You can lose fat without losing weight, especially if you're building shapely muscle through strength training, nutraplenishing, and eating "clean" food and drinking "clean" water. And since muscle weighs more than twice as much as fat, it's quite possible to lose fat without shedding a significant amount of weight.

What's insidious about calorie-deprivation diets is that all the self-denial and misapplied willpower that you manage to summon up often ends up costing you muscle mass, which is the last thing you want. You lose weight all right, but it's the wrong weight. The price of rapid weight loss is compromised health and a gaunt, emaciated look if you keep it up long enough. But, of course, you can't keep starving yourself forever. And when you do gain the weight back, and you will *always* gain it back eventually, do you think it's in the form of replaced muscle mass? Not likely, my friend. Unfortunately, it's all fat. You'll end up with more body fat than you started with, even when you are in the reduced-weight phase. That's why veteran yo-yo dieters begin nutraplenishing with lower VHI scores. They're starting off handicapped, like a weighted-down horse in a race. But if you're one of those veteran yo-yo dieters, don't despair. Most people come to the Nashville Diet after not one but several cracks at the fad-diet flavor of the month. It's the norm. You're like the great heroes of mythology who are led astray and so must first fight the dragons before discovering the true path. You've tried it their way and paid the price. Now it's time to get healthy and lean for good.

SHED FAT BY EATING, NOT BY STARVING

Yo-yo diets that depend on calorie deprivation (a fancy term for starving yourself thin) are guilty of another sin. When you deprive your body of calories your body will instinctively switch into starvation mode by turning your metabolism down a couple of notches. When that happens, it concentrates on conserving body fat because that's your "emergency back-up" to sustain life. Your body's first priority is survival, and starvation mode is classic survival logic. "It looks like I'm not going to be getting the energy I need for a long time," your body tells itself. "So I'm going to hang on to the best emergency energy source I've got (body fat)."

Need I point out that this is counterproductive, to put it mildly? Yet I've met very few people with body fat problems who haven't tried to willpower their way to leanness by starving their cells instead of nourishing them. They never imagine that by doing so they're actually discouraging their body from letting go of fat and slowly but surely turning their metabolism down. They're also condemning themselves to failure, since it's literally impossible to starve yourself for very long. And when that yo-yo comes back up, it always comes back higher.

It gets worse. We've talked about metabolism, remember? The key point here is that your metabolic rate (that is, the efficiency with which your body processes food) is heavily influenced by your fat-to-lean-muscle ratio. As you lose more muscle mass than fat as a result of yo-yo dieting, your metabolic rate suffers proportionally. A lower metabolic rate decreases the number of calories your body can handle before giving up and storing them away as fat. So even with your reduced food intake, you're creating fat faster. The more you starve yourself, the more sluggish your metabolic rate will be, and the more calories will be converted to fat. Meanwhile, of course, your appetite is growing, not shrinking, and creating cravings for precisely the quick-energy foods you must stay away from even when you're eating normally. Once you (inevitably) give in to those cravings and end your self-imposed virtual fast, your compromised metabolism will be overwhelmed and much less able to handle the flood of calories than it was when you started. You'll soon be fatter than ever, less healthy than ever, and more in need of nutraplenishing than ever.

Starving your body has one more unhealthy mechanism. Since your body is holding on to your fat so tightly, your body gets totally confused and starts burning lean muscle for calories, for the energy it needs.

So, to recap: When you're not nutraplenishing *and* you put your body in starvation mode, here's what happens: You decrease your metabolism, burn up lean muscle mass, and gain more fat as a percentage of your body, which decreases your metabolism even further and increases your appetite, which means you'll eventually be eating and gaining back the "weight," only this time it will be all fat. You can actually end up back at the same weight, only much "fatter," with a lower metabolism yet. None of this depressing vicious cycle applies with the program you're getting here. I'm going to make sure of that by insisting that you adhere to two mandatory edicts: you must eat and you must not weigh yourself!

You have to eat! The Nashville Diet is not a calorie-deprivation diet, not a yo-yo diet, not even a "diet" at all in the traditional sense of food restriction. Rather than deprive, it provides. What it provides is the nutrients your cells need. As you replenish your nutrients, your appetite will, in time, revert to a healthy level. Skipping meals is forbidden. On the contrary, your success will depend on regular healthy meals that keep your metabolism stoked. Yes, you will eat less than you have been, because your nutraplenishing will reduce your cravings. Yes, you will eat differently than you have been, because you'll be replacing processed and other toxic foods with their naturally healthy "live" equivalents. And you'll be eating less often than before because your cells will be satisfied enough not to pester your appetite between meals. But you *will* eat. And you'll enjoy it. That's an order!

Stay off the scales! Weighing yourself every day leads to three things: confusion, discouragement, and deception. I've already explained how you can lose weight without losing fat or gaining health. And I've explained how you can be making great progress that doesn't necessarily move the needle much.

Millions of Americans make the tragic mistake of assuming they're getting permanently lean and healthy because their scale tells them so. It would be equally tragic to abandon a sure-fire route to true vibrant health and a perfect body fat percentage just because you don't think a needle is moving enough.

If you feel healthier, look better, and are wearing clothes you couldn't have dreamed of wearing before, what difference does it make what your scale says?!? The *only numbers that matter* are your clothes size, body fat percentage (and almost any gym can measure that for you—usually at no charge), and your VHI.

I'll let you in on a little secret. Now that I have recovered my vibrant health through nutraplenishing, I wear the same dress size I wore in high school, even though I weigh twenty pounds more! A miracle? No. It's the result of a tuned, humming metabolism, along with the excellent fat-to-lean-muscle ratio *that I never had in high school.*

Rest assured that when the needle does move down after you've followed this program faithfully, it will be for a greater good. At 5'9", I would shrink maybe one dress size for every ten pounds I lost on typical diets. ABut as I used what eventually became the Nashville Diet to recover from my illness, I shrank five dress sizes while losing just twenty-five pounds. That's the kind of cost-effective weight loss that you want! So don't weigh yourself more than once a week for the purposes of updating your VHI. I'd even recommend weighing yourself less often than that, and simply "guesstimating" your weight for the VHI for those weeks you don't weigh yourself. You won't be off by all that much. Do yourself a favor. Hide your scale in a hard-to-reach corner of the closet and only pull it out every one to four weeks. And when you do use it, don't make a big deal out of it, one way or the other. The Nashville Diet is about how you look and feel, not a needle position.

THE ONLY STRATEGIES YOU NEED

The principal strategy of the Nashville Diet is to take your nutrients faithfully. That health-giving habit, along with the more aggressive detoxification regimen it leads to, restores your internal balance so that you can more easily stop overeating and switch to the kinds of foods that allow you to achieve your fat-loss goals. While *what* you eat is the most important "diet" element in the program, I've found that two additional strategies— separation and rotation, which deal with *how* you eat, are extremely helpful.

SEPARATION

Space your three meals four to five hours apart. I believe in the time-honored tradition of eating three square meals a day. You will not be switching to five "mini-meals" a day, or incorporating midmorning and midafternoon snacks into your eating schedule. I know the vogue these days is to eat more and smaller meals. And there are merits in that approach for people whose systems are balanced enough to support a high metabolic rate. But it's not right for somebody who's trying to restore internal balance by embarking on a cell-nourishing program. First of all, there's simply no need to add another layer of change to your life. You're already taking a fistful of capsules twice a day. You're also incorporating detox exercises into your routine, starting cardiovascular and strength training, and concentrating on bringing nontoxic live food to the table. Rearranging your meal schedule on top of all that is overkill.

Also, to be honest, the whole idea of sanctioning between-meal eating offers too many temptations to a recovering crave-slave. That so-called light healthy mid-afternoon snack can easily turn into an excuse for indulging in sugary sweets for old time's sake. Much better to treat yourself to a satisfying meal of live food and then forget about eating until the next meal.

After any meal, always wait at least four hours before eating again, but no longer than five. You need this "separation" to give your body time to burn some stored fat for fuel rather than just the readily available energy from the last meal. If you eat every time you feel the slightest hunger, your body never has the time to burn fat for fuel. Wait four hours instead, but don't wait longer than five. If you extend the separation any longer, your blood sugar will crash while your appetite soars through the roof. Next thing you know, you're craving sugar again, which is precisely the problem you've worked so hard to overcome. So except while you're sleeping, of course, plan your meals no more than five hours apart.

This four- to five-hour separation plan should accommodate your usual three-meal schedule, with perhaps just slight modifications. If you're used to eating breakfast at 7 A.M. and lunch at 1 P.M., you're going to have to shift one or both to get that six-hour separation down to five. You might have to eat dinner a little earlier than you have been (which is never a bad idea anyway). Meals at 8 A.M., 1 P.M., and 6 P.M., for example, should pose no problem to your eating schedule.

What if you find yourself feeling hungry before four hours have passed? Don't panic. And don't run to the refrigerator. Instead, ask yourself how hungry you really are. Frankly, I always tell my clients that a little bit of hunger never hurt anybody. There's a difference between starving yourself and not giving in to every little hunger pang that decides to rear its head. Your nutrients are working hard to restore your appetite to normal and quash cravings. Why not help them out a little along the way?

Try drinking plenty of water. Untimely hunger is often your body's code language for thirst. Let your first reaction to between-meal hunger be a 16-ounce glass of clean, cool water. If your body is positively screaming for food every two or three hours, adjust the meals you eat at the proper time rather than snack between meals. Your portions probably need to be slightly higher. Increase the protein in those meals, and see what effect that has on your between-meal hunger pangs.

If you're feeling famished before a meal because you waited more than five hours, you can take some preventive action. Instead of feasting in a way you'll regret, fight fire with fire by having just a bit of dessert *first*. By taking just a few bites of something sweet (just a few bites, mind you) and drinking a glass of water, you can get your blood sugar back up without overindulging. Then go ahead and have your usual, moderate meal (even if you no longer feel like eating it). This little "pre-ssert" isn't something you want to make a habit of, but it can occasionally serve as damage control when you put off eating for more than five hours.

ROTATION

Rotation is all about tricking your metabolism. After you've felt the bene-fits of your nutraplenishing and detox efforts, and you've made good progress on your transition from toxic food to live food, you can make quicker fat-loss progress by employing a modified version of what's called rotation dieting.

The concept is simple: You allow yourself brief periods of very-low-calorie eating so your body can burn maximum amounts of fat. These will be your "fat-burning" days. But you quickly return to your full portions be-fore your body's metabolism reacts by slowing down. These will be your "full eating" days. (Of course, those full portions are your new, smaller full portions, not the oversized version of the old days.) Go about this by eating half your usual amount for four days of the week. For the other three, eat as you normally do. Coordinate this calorie-intake rotation with your rota-tion of the Masters of Metabolism category of nutrients. Your three full-food days will be the same three days that you don't take the full complement of those Masters. Rotate for no more than four weeks at a time.

I don't like to talk much about calories. For one thing, I've found that it causes more confusion than anything else. I prefer you to find your best food-intake level naturally as your nutraplenishing stabilizes your appetite. But here I'll mention calories to illustrate this metabolism-tricking concept of rotation dieting.

A simple rule of thumb for the approximate number of calories you need to maintain your weight at a certain level is to take the weight you think you want to be and add a zero to it. If you think you want to weight 130 pounds, then you would consume 1,300 calories a day to maintain that weight. Of course, you don't really know what you want to weigh, but this way you'll at least have a guide.

In theory, you would speed up your fat loss by eating 1,300 calories on Friday, Saturday, and Sunday, and cutting that in half to 650 calories on your four low-calorie days. Now, if you weigh 200 pounds right now and are used to eating more than 2,000 calories a day, it would be an act of utter madness to try to eat just 1,300 calories a day, let alone 650. Don't even consider it. You'd be creating a train wreck by jamming on the brakes while going 150 miles an hour. Instead, allow time for your nutraplenishing to get your daily calorie intake slowly down to something within shouting distance of your calorie goal (say, 1,600). Then take it down in increments along the lines of 25 percent less each week for the four weeks. So when you're ready to do some rotation dieting, you might eat 1,600 calories Friday through Sunday of the first week, and 800 the other four days. The next week you can try for 1,500 on the full days and 750 on the rotation days. By the fourth week, you may be able to reach your goal of 1,300, with 650 your limit on rotation days.

If this much calorie restriction seems like too much for you at this point, then either you're not on the right high-quality nutrients, you're not consuming the correct amounts, or you haven't been on them in full doses for at least thirty days.

Mike's story. I met Mike and Kim, a sweet couple from Phoenix, Arizona, under unusual circumstances. Mike wanted *Kim* to get on the Nashville Diet program for health reasons, but Kim felt it more important for *Mike* to get on the program for the same reasons. *They both wanted to* *get back to their premarriage weight.* So after counseling them both, I got them started on the nutrients at the same time.

It was so gratifying to hear both of them tell what the nutrients and program were doing in each of their lives. Mike said he was feeling *much* better, but could never see his own eating habits coming under control. In the meantime, I had the opportunity to eat with both of them on several occasions. Mike's eating habits were the worst! He routinely consumed three to four large sodas with each meal. The caloric intake and volume of each of his meals was astonishing, and he would eat everything put before him.

After being on the nutrients for exactly thirty days, Mike called me. He *tried* to continue to eat as much, but couldn't do it! "I can only eat half as much!" he said. And he *felt better.* "Last night I could only drink a half of a Coke with dinner, and that was only out of habit; I didn't really want it. I've been like this for about two weeks, but I haven't lost any weight," he said. I just wanted to bonk him on the head! Of course he hadn't lost any weight yet—that's not the idea. He now has to keep it going long enough to build some lean muscle back and restart his metabolism.

So you see that the idea is to wait until you instinctively *want* to eat less and eat different foods. *Only then* do you reduce the amount and change the types of foods that you eat. This process, once started, will keep you coming back.

Rotation dieting helps you pick up the pace after you've already started moving up the VHI scale. Don't ever go more than four days at the reduced-calorie level or you'll cross the line to metabolism-crashing yo-yo dieting. Make sure you eat healthy portions on your full-calorie days. And don't prolong your rotation dieting in the hopes of short cutting your way to leanness. Your long-term vibrant health will be the result of the consistent good eating habits you've developed by nutraplenishing, detoxing, and focusing on live food.

Keep it up and that fat's going to melt away before your very eyes!

lean for life

imagine yourself three, six, maybe twelve or eighteen months from now. You're enjoying life with an energy you haven't experienced since you were a child. You're feeling wonderful inside, knowing that decades of accumulated toxins have been flushed from your cells and your once-undernourished systems are functioning on all cylinders. You're focused and aware as you walk through the world, controlling your environment to avoid the poisons that most people constantly absorb unawares.

You're consuming almost all live food and you wonder how you ever were able to eat the toxin-riddled processed food of your past. Your weight is where you want it to be, your wardrobe is completely new (since your old clothes are way too big), and when you look in the mirror you like what you see. You've faithfully followed the Nashville Diet and now you're reaping the rewards.

You feel great. You look great. You *are* great.

So would your next step then be to say to yourself, "Okay, that's enough if this! I've done my job. Now I'm going back to my old life"? Probably not, I venture to say. But almost everybody on typical fad diets do end up going back and they go back long before they're anywhere close to achieving the results that you will. By definition, calorie deprivation is temporary. By its nature, it cannot lead to vibrant health. What you're doing is different. In fact, it's the total opposite.

The goal of the Nashville Diet is to restore your overall health, permanently. The weight loss you'll experience is the *result* of better health, not a prerequisite for it. I have consistently seen that when my clients start looking healthier and feeling more energetic, they find it surprisingly easy to reach and then maintain their healthy weight.

But here's what's really important for you. My successful clients develop a strong tendency to continue the healthy ways they've adopted. As a Nashville Diet graduate, you will too. You won't feel like you've "given up" anything. Instead, you'll feel like you've found what you were looking for. Vibrant health is forever.

KEEP TAKING YOUR NUTRIENTS

Say we lived in a perfect world. A world where the foods we eat deliver the natural nutrients they're supposed to. After eating three healthy, natural, cell-nourishing meals a day for a year, would it make sense to stop eating after that because you've already been nourished? No way. We need to feed our cells continuously, every day for our entire lives. Obvious, isn't it? Yet I can't tell you how many clients have asked me at some point when they can stop taking their nutrients. Since we'll never get the nutrients we need from our food supply, the answer is always the same: Never! Supplementation with nutraceuticals is not something you do temporarily while you're "on a diet." It is a lifetime strategy for vibrant health and a lean, fit body. This is why I so often encourage you to think of your nutrients as food—which is what they are. You don't stop eating, do you? Nor do you stop taking nutrients—unless, of course, you don't mind going back to the way you were before you had vibrant health.

Some of my clients who have made significant progress word the question differently. They have a new internal health and energy and have dropped several sizes, so they feel that they've reached the point where they're now completely "nutraplenished." There are also some clients who feel that way but have *not* made much progress, because they're not following the program. But they still insist they're already "nutraplenished."

Here's my response to that. While there's never going to be a time where you don't need to keep feeding your cells with the Nashville Diet nutraceuticals, you will reach a point where your strategy shifts to "maintenance." In other words, your weight is where you want it to be, your VHI is in the 90s, and you've implemented all the diet and exercise recommendations I've given you. Here's where you're ready to scale back your nutrient regimen, without eliminating it.

Cut back on your nutrient dosages the same way you built them up — gradually, one nutrient group at a time. Start from the last nutrient group and work toward the first. For example, when you feel you're ready, take your dosage of the Detox Delights down one notch. Try it at the new dosage for a few days and see if you notice any negative changes in your eating habits, bodily functions, or just in the way you feel.

If all's fine and dandy, cut back on your Masters of Metabolism and make the same observations. This will be a trial-and-error process. Tweak away at the dosages until you've found the minimum level of each nutrient group that doesn't jeopardize your newfound health. The beauty of it is that by this time, you're so in touch with your less toxic (and thinner) body that you can monitor its changes effectively. You're calling the shots now, not the toxins or the cravings.

Another adjustment you can make with your nutrients once you're lean and healthy is in the timing. With a little experimentation, you may find that taking one nutrient group later in the day keeps you cravings-free a little bit more efficiently. (Don't, however, take the Masters of Metabolism past lunchtime.) You'll also find that you can take advantage of your nutrients by adjusting them to specific situations. If you're exposed accidentally to a strong toxin source, find yourself cheating on your foods too much, or are on your way to a social situation where the alcohol and snacks flow freely, grab those capsule bottles and take a full, morning dose of everything *before* you are tempted. Many veteran Nashville Dieters get to know their nutrients and bodies so well that they can tailor "emergency" doses of certain nutrients to fit different situations.

Remember though, that adjusting nutrient intake is the privilege of the successful followers of the program who are at the maintenance stage. Until you have completely reached your goals, don't try to adjust your nutrients by reducing your intake. Don't stop because you think you no longer need them. And don't stop because you're discouraged at the early stages. If you take your nutrients and follow the program, you *will* get results. If you keep taking your nutrients and continue to follow the program, you will continue to enjoy those results forever. If you stop taking your nutrients for any reason, you *will* regress. That's how powerful these nutraceuticals are. You've found the key to success. Don't throw it away.

THE BODY IMBALANCE

Eliminating toxic foods from your diet and replacing them with live food is what the "diet" aspect of the Nashville Diet program is all about. But once you've made the transition from processed food to live food, you may want to start paying attention to which combinations of live foods will best help you achieve your health and weight goals. Do this by selecting foods that will offset the imbalances in your system resulting from your body type.

If you're like most people whose weight is too high and health too low, your body is dominated by one of four hormone-producing organs: the adrenal glands, the pituitary gland, the ovaries, or the thyroid. The excess hormones released by an overactive gland lead to cravings for certain foods, dictate where fat is apportioned, and create imbalances that work against your goals of nourishing cells, flushing out toxins, and shedding body fat. Your body imbalance is determined by which gland is overactive and dominating your individual system. The strategy to overcome that imbalance is to stimulate some organs while resting the overworked one by emphasizing certain foods in the diet.

Adapting the work of such pioneers as Henry Bieler, M.D., and Elliot D. Abravanel, M.D., I've come up with some recommendations for eating to balance your body as you follow our nutraplenishing and detoxification strategies.

These recommendations are not for an open-ended lifetime eating program. They can't be permanent because they depend on imbalance to achieve balance. In other words, these eating guidelines are exaggerated in one direction to offset your body type's exaggerated imbalance in the other direction. You'll even find instances of breaking some of the taboos in the food choice guidelines outlined in Chapter Ten. So use these body type guidelines solely for the purpose of achieving balance. They're temporary. Once you achieve balance—which you'll recognize by your rising VHI and shrinking waistline—you can put these recommendations aside in favor of eating regular meals (of live, unprocessed food, of course), and by adhering to all the healthy eating strategies you learned in the last three chapters.

WHAT'S YOUR BODY IMBALANCE?

Your first order of business is to determine your body imbalance. That is, which of the four organs is your body predisposed to favor? Which of these four—adrenals, thyroid, pituitaries, or ovaries—is dominant enough to demand extra "hits" of certain problem foods, resulting in addictive food cravings and accumulations of body fat in specific areas?

The answer will tell you which of the "tribes of Imbalancium" you belong to. Are you an "adrenalite," with overactive adrenal glands? A "pituitarian," with overactive pituitary glands? Perhaps a gonadite, with overactive ovaries? Or are you a "thyroidian," with overactive thyroids?

Let's take a look at the characteristics of each body imbalance. Choose the one that suits you most closely, referring to your journal entries over the weeks for clues. Then we'll see what eating guidelines will set things straight.

The Adrenalites

The extra adrenaline in your system may make you feel powerful and slow to tire. Nothing wrong with that, is there? The problem is that because this feeling is now the norm with you, you rely on it too much and overeat the foods that activate your already overactive adrenal glands. You tend to crave fatty foods, salt, red meat, and eggs. Adrenalites enjoy fermented things, like alcohol, because such foods really give them the hormonal "high" they've become addicted to. It's not unusual for an adrenalite to eat three hearty, protein-laden meals, and then throw in some salty snacks like salted nuts, salami, or aged cheese. Adrenalites don't mind skipping dessert, but they must have their red wine or after-dinner drink!

As the adrenalite becomes more malnourished, they begin to exhaust their adrenals; consequently, more imbalanced weight tends to be deposited in the belly. Men will assume a capital "D" shape. Women who are adrenal aren't prone to cellulite, but they will carry weight in their belly, even as their legs stay shapely and slender.

The Gonadites

These are women whose ovaries are dominating their metabolism, while their thyroid and pituitary glands get shortchanged. Result: Constant exhaustion and fat accumulation in the rear and outer thighs. Of all the body types, a gonadite is the most susceptible to cellulite. Her stomach is fairly flat, but she's carrying saddlebags on the outside of her legs. An imbalanced gonadite will be noticeably pear-shaped. The ovaries are stimulated by spice, grease, and alcohol. For this reason, most gonads crave these things. Mexican food is a major problem for gonadites, as are many other spicy ethnic foods. Gonadites also crave rich sauces, creamy dips, and dishes made with cheese or butter.

The Pituitarians

There's a close association between dairy products and pituitary function. The hormone prolactin in mother's milk stimulates the baby's pituitary activity, promoting brain development. Not surprisingly, adult pituitarians crave milk and milk products like cheese, yogurt, ice cream, and cream- or cheese-based sauces. They also usually love pizza, peanut butter, and pickles. A balanced pituitarian will often boast a sensual shape and youthful appearance, with a straight neck, trim body, and well-rounded bottom. For the unbalanced pituitary type, it's a different story. "Baby fat" will apportion itself throughout the body, rather than in a few spots like the thighs or tummy. Their digestion is often poor (because their adrenal glands are overwhelmed by the pituitary) and their libido is low (because their ovaries are also overwhelmed by the pituitary).

The Thyroidians

The overactive thyroid tends to produce quick bursts of energy separated by down periods. A thyroidian craves that zippy feeling, and seeks it through sweet or starchy carbohydrates—sweet foods, bread, and pasta. They're sugar seekers and caffeine takers. For them, even fruit is really a sugar fix, because of the fructose fruit offers. Thyroidians tend to be long-limbed and slender-waisted. When out of balance, they'll often be burdened with cellulite on the thighs, hips, and upper arms, even if they're not particularly overweight. The lack of tone in their muscles makes them sag.

YOUR BODY TYPE FOOD PLAN

Do you recognize your body type in one of the four descriptions? Or (as sometimes happens) did you see yourself in two of them? If so, use a little trial and error. Re-read the descriptions, concentrating only on the cravings, and pick the body type that most closely describes your cravings. Follow the food guidelines for that body type for a month. If there's little change, switch to the other type that seemed to describe you.

It's possible you see yourself in all or none of the body types. If so, go through the types again, concentrating first on the cravings, then on body features. See if you can narrow it down. If not, consider yourself a member of the neutral tribe. This is often the case for those who are more than 30 pounds overweight or with a VHI under 70. If that's you, focus on your nutrients and the general food guidelines. Then take another look at the body type list each month as you make progress. When you're ready to try a food program for your body imbalance, one of the following programs will help you get to your weight loss goals at a faster rate.

Food Program for Adrenalites

Since your previous eating patterns have overstimulated your adrenals, your strategy is to balance your endocrine (hormonal) system by eating to gently stimulate your thyroid and pituitary glands. To do that, you must avoid red meat, full-fat cheese, greasy food, and salt during this body type phase of your program. Get your protein from fish, chicken, legumes, tofu, and light dairy products like cottage cheese, yogurt, and nonfat milk. You want to eat a small breakfast of whole-grain cereal or dairy. Your lunch should also be light (salad, cooked vegetables, dairy, fish, or fruit). Adrenalites can make dinner their heaviest meal. It should consist of chicken or fish, legumes (beans, etc.), vegetables, and fruit. Beware of late afternoon hunger. You may be able to get past it if you drink hot parsley tea, with a small amount of honey or sugar. If you absolutely must snack between lunch and dinner, make it a small yogurt and a half a glass of skim milk.

ADRENALITE FOOD COMPONENT BREAKDOWN

80 PERCENT	Whole grains, fresh fruit and vegetables, legumes (beans, etc.), and/or low-fat dairy
20 PERCENT	Refined grains (like white rice), vegetable oils, small amounts of sugar or caffeine, and lighter proteins (eggs, chicken, and fish)

O PERCENT   Red meat or shellfish, alcohol, salt, creamy or buttery
             dishes, full-fat cheeses. Avoid these foods completely.

ADRENALITE MENU SUGGESTIONS

Meal	Fat-Burning Days	Full Eating Days
BREAKFAST (7:30 A.M.)	1 cup fruit salad w/yogurt	Organic oats w/blueberries or cranberries, 1 slice 12-grain bread
LUNCH (I I:30 A.M.)	Large Caesar salad, 12-grain bread cheese sandwich	2 cups navy beans, 1 slice 12-grain bread, Large Caesar salad
SNACK (4:30 P.M.)	1 Pear (organically grown)	1 Apple (organically grown)
DINNER (6:30 P.M.)	¼ cup Breyers® ice cream w/fresh or frozen mixed berries (organically grown)	Large mixed greens salad, ½ chicken breast (free range)

Food Program for Gonadites

Your strategy is to gently stimulate your thyroid and pituitary glands and
calm your ovaries to balance out your system. Emphasize fruit. Gonadites
are one group that can benefit from a temporary semi-vegetarian diet. If
you want to try stopping all meat for a month or so, your best source of
protein would be eggs, legumes, tofu, and light dairy products. Cottage
cheese and low-fat yogurt are particularly good for you, since they gently
stimulate your lagging organs.

Keep your breakfast very light—as little as a piece of fruit and some
herbal tea (red clover is best for you). Keep your lunch light as well and
let dinner be your heaviest meal. That will cut down on evening snack
cravings. Late morning will also be a troubling time for you. Drink hot red
clover tea if you're feeling hunger pangs when you shouldn't. A tiny bit of
honey or sugar in it is okay. If you succumb to a snack, it should be fruit,
like a few grapes or strawberries.

GONADITE FOOD COMPONENT BREAKDOWN

80 PERCENT   Dairy products, fresh fruit and vegetables, whole grains, legumes (beans, etc.)

20 PERCENT   Limited carbohydrates (mostly from whole grains) and light proteins like eggs, chicken, fish, or tofu.

0 PERCENT   Red meat, stimulating spices, creamy dishes, buttery dishes, greasy dishes, and alcohol. Avoid these foods completely.

GONADITE MENU SUGGESTIONS

Meal	Fat-Burning Days	Full Eating Days
BREAKFAST (7:30 A.M.)	2 cups fruit salad w/yogurt	Whole grain organic cereal w/blueberries (fresh or frozen organically grown), 1 slice 7-grain toast
LUNCH (11:30 A.M.)	2 cups vegetable soup (homemade, organically grown)	Full plate of vegetable(s) of your choice, 1 slice multigrain bread, 1 cup plain yogurt w/fresh fruit (organically grown)
SNACK (4:30 P.M.)	1 Apple (organically grown)	1 pear (organically grown)
DINNER (6:30 P.M.)	½ slice multigrain bread, 1 cup navy beans	2 cups pinto beans, 1 cup quinoa or long-grain rice, large serving of steamed cauliflower

Food Program for Pituitarians

You need high protein, low carbohydrate, no dairy, and no caffeine or sugar. High protein means plenty of beef and organ meats, with chicken and fish thrown in for variety. Low carbohydrate means no sugar, a min-

imum of fruit, and moderate amounts of whole grain. Emphasize cooked
or raw fresh vegetables over fruit.

Your biggest meal needs to be breakfast—never skip it. And cereal
isn't appropriate for a pituitarian breakfast. Have a meat serving, something like 4 ounces of calves' liver, along with a half slice of whole grain
toast and a cup of decaf. Your lunch will be moderate—try 4 ounces of
fish or chicken and steamed vegetables. Dinner will be lighter still, with
maybe a light meat and a salad or cooked vegetable. Your danger time is
late afternoon, when you may crave cheese or yogurt or sweets. Resist the
temptation at all costs. Try drinking hot fenugreek tea, without sugar. If
you must snack, have a few bites of meat.

PITUITARIAN FOOD COMPONENT BREAKDOWN

80 PERCENT	Red meat, organ meat, pork, lamb, eggs, poultry, fish, shellfish, and fresh vegetables
20 PERCENT	Some butter, some vegetable oil, legumes (beans, etc.), whole grains, some fresh fruit, and oat milk or rice milk
0 PERCENT	Dairy, caffeine, sugar, refined grains. Avoid these foods completely.

PITUITARIAN MENU SUGGESTIONS

Meal	Fat-Burning Days	Full Eating Days
BREAKFAST (7:30 A.M.)	2 eggs (free-range organic)	1 pork chop, 1 egg
LUNCH (11:30 A.M.)	1 slice roast beef, 1 cup vegetable medley	1 steak, 2 cups of any vegetable(s)
SNACK (4:30 P.M.)	¼ chicken breast (free range)	Handful of raw nuts of your choice
DINNER (6:30 P.M.)	1 cup raw cauliflower and broccoli	Roast beef sandwich with mustard, mixed greens, and sliced tomatoes, on 12-grain bread

Food Program for Thyroidians

Most important for thyroidians is the timing of your eating. You need to steady your energy and reduce the sugar racing and cravings from all that thyroid output. Cling hard to our separation rule (four hours between meals but never more than five). All three meals should be more or less of the same size. Never skip breakfast. Your danger times vary. Thyroid stimulation drops your blood sugar levels, making you crave sweets. You can try raspberry herb tea (no sugar or honey) to beat your afternoon cravings. If that fails, snack on half a hard-boiled egg, or two or three bites of chicken or fish. In your meals, get lots of protein from chicken and fish, but go easy on the red meat. Light dairy (cottage cheese, yogurt, and nonfat milk) is okay for added protein. Eat eggs every day. Sugar (including fruit) and starchy carbohydrates must be avoided in favor of whole grain and lots of fresh vegetables.

THYROIDIAN FOOD COMPONENT BREAKDOWN

80 PERCENT	Eggs, poultry, fish and shellfish, low-fat dairy
20 PERCENT	Some red meat, vegetable oil, some butter, legumes (beans, etc.), and whole grain
0 PERCENT	Refined grains, starchy carbohydrates (white rice, potatoes, pasta, white bread, crackers), caffeine, sugar, and fruit. Avoid these foods completely.

THYROIDIAN MENU SUGGESTIONS

Meal	Fat-Burning Days	Full Eating Days
BREAKFAST (7:30 A.M.)	1 Hard-boiled egg (free-range organic)	Hot grain cereal
LUNCH (11:30 A.M.)	Grilled chicken salad: ½ chicken breast (free range), mostly lettuce—romaine and/or mesclun greens	Grilled chicken salad: ½ chicken breast (free range), mostly lettuce—romaine and/or mesclun greens, 4 spears steamed broccoli

Meal	Fat-Burning Days	Full Eating Days
SNACK (4:30 P.M.)	½ cup raw broccoli and cauliflower sprinkled with balsamic vinegar	1 Hard-boiled egg (free range organic)
DINNER (6:30 P.M.)	1 cup vegetable medley soup (home-made; organically grown)	Salmon steak, steamed squash or zucchini and onions drizzled with 2 table-spoons olive oil, fresh lemon juice, and Herbamare*

*Herbamare is a seasoning made with sea salt and 14 herbs, and marketed by Rapunzel Pure Organics, Inc.

VIBRANT HEALTH IS FOREVER

The Nashville Diet cannot fail.

How can I can make such a bold statement? Because the Nashville Diet's purpose is to restore cellular health. Every time you take your nutrients, you are, without fail, restoring the health of your cells. With every toxic particle you flush from your system, you're restoring the health of your cells. And every bite of live food that replaces processed food restores health to your cells. Your newfound health from following this program represents an astounding success. And you *will* lose your excess body fat because your nutraplenishing, detox regimen, and healthy eating go right to the roots of your weight problems.

There are, however, two roads that lead to failure. One is paved with impatience. It's taken by those who expect that a lifetime of nutrient depletion and toxic accumulation is going to disappear after a week of taking magic capsules. This is the get-rich-quick mentality that fuels the diet industry. Do not allow yourself to be a victim of it again. It appeals to those who prefer to see the scales move *now* rather than dedicate themselves to going to the root cause of their weight and health problems to solve them once and for all. Those folks will not find what they want in this program.

The other road to failure is paved with discouragement. You will experience setbacks as you work to restore your vibrant health. You will backslide on your food habits. You'll succumb to a craving now and then. You
might even forget to take your nutrients with you on vacation and miss a
week of cell nourishment. Everyone stumbles. But not everyone deals
with setbacks equally. Some make it very hard, get discouraged, and either
abandon their health and fat-loss goals or start "improvising" in unhelpful
ways. Others pick themselves up, dust themselves off, and move ahead
with renewed determination.

I and the counselors at my clinic spend a lot of our time helping
clients work their way through the inevitable setbacks and come out
stronger on the other side. I'd like to spend the rest of this chapter helping
you do the same thing.

PATIENCE IS YOUR SOURCE OF STRENGTH AND SUCCESS

The most important piece of advice I can give you is to be clear about
your mission going in. You're not in this to "lose weight" quickly. You're
in it to lose weight *permanently* by restoring your internal health. It may
be a month or three months before you weigh less than you did when you
started. On the other hand, it may be a week. It doesn't matter! You're
making progress all the while. Throw away the scales and be patient!

As you know well by now, the Nashville Diet moves along in three
phases. First you nutraplenish. Then you actively detoxify your system and
surroundings. Then—and only then—you start changing your eating
habits. This might not come until your third month on the program. And
the limited amount of more aggressive dieting on the program—such as
rotation dieting—can only be done after time is spent on those first three
stages. Health first! Weight loss follows.

So if you're looking to fit into your high school prom dress in time for
the reunion next month, you've come to the wrong place! On the other
hand, if you want to steadily start feeling better, looking better, and
moving toward your best weight (and then staying at that weight perma-

nently) put on your patience cap, put those nutrients in your mouth, and swallow!

A number of other factors in the Nashville Diet plan can require even more patience. Here are the most common, and some suggestions for how to overcome them.

A low VHI. When you start out with a VHI in the 50s or lower, you'll have to move ahead more slowly. You need to follow the nutraplenishing instructions in Chapter Four to get your VHI up to 70 before graduating to detox and beyond. But please don't be discouraged. That low VHI number really only confirms what you were already feeling and seeing about yourself. And since the main focus of this program is addressing weight problems through improved health, you have the most benefits to gain in the early stages. You're doing the right thing!

A long history. If you're fifty and you've been overweight and/or sick since you were a teenager, it's simply going to take you longer to build up your long-depressed systems. Many people in your situation cannot just detox from existing healthy cells; they actually have to build new ones. That takes time. But it gets done if you stick with it. You've waited thirty years to turn things around. Now I'm asking you to wait just a few extra months.

Yo-yo dieting history. You learned in the last chapter how fast weight loss followed by inevitable weight gain compromises your metabolism. That puts you in a deeper hole coming into the Nashville Diet, so don't be surprised if your results come slowly. It may be 90 days before you cash in with noticeable weight loss, but I promise you'll feel steadily better and more energetic as you work toward that goal.

BREAKING THROUGH THOSE LOGJAMS

While patience is usually the answer to any perceived delay in your progress from fat to lean, sometimes there really are identifiable problems that hold you back. If your VHI is 70 or higher, you should feel great about your progress by the ninety-day mark. If not, something might be amiss. Let's look at the main possible roadblocks that we can move aside.

Are you faithful to your nutrients? The nutrient regimen outlined in Chapter Four is the result of much research and clinical application. It is carefully designed to do the job. You must take the full complement of capsules every day to get results. And you must increase the dosages to maximum according to the schedule given. I know that's a lot of pills to swallow, but the payoff is worth it. If you skimp on your nutraplenishing, you'll undermine the entire program. So take your capsules without fail!

Are you doing everything else? Not much of the instruction I've given you up to now is optional. "You gotta" do it all. Some of our clients pick and choose their way through the program and then wonder why it "doesn't work." But of course, you can't say a program doesn't work if you don't follow it. So, are you practicing the detox techniques? Are you starting to exercise? To help you remember to do everything, you'll find a complete week-by-week checklist of your duties in Chapter Thirteen. Follow it to the letter and you'll love the results.

Are you improvising? This is sometimes a stumbling block with yo-yo diet veterans. They've internalized so much "diet" advice that they sometimes like to throw in their favorites where they don't belong. One night they just may discard the Nashville Diet eating guidelines and gorge themselves on some toxic food and justify it because some other diet says it's okay. Is that you? If so, no wonder your progress is slow or nonexistent! Please don't freelance. You've tried it their way. Now try it the Nashville way—to the letter.

Are you eating? If you skip meals, you're not helping your cause. You must eat regular meals. And you must avoid the all-or-nothing mentality. One client called me one afternoon proud of herself because all she'd had that day was a cup of coffee and an ice cream sandwich. Need I point out that skipping meals and then putting caffeine and sugar in your body is not at all what the Nashville Diet is all about?

Are you being exposed to toxins? There is a tendency for anybody on the program to hit what I call the toxic wall. That's simply a point where the toxins just aren't breaking loose from your fat cells as much. There can be lots of reasons for this. Most of the time, it's a matter of working though this stage, making sure you're getting your exercise, performing your detox techniques, and taking your nutrients. But also check for new sources of toxic exposure or previously undetected sources. When my clients hit the wall, we often trace the problem to mold or other toxic sources. Another possibility is your ongoing pharmaceutical intake. Don't stop it on your own, but consult your doctor about the possibility of getting off the medication.

SETTIN' STRAIGHT YOUR CHEATIN' HEART

If human beings threw in the towel after every setback, we'd still be living in caves. But we're blessed with a drive to overcome obstacles to reach our goals. You need to apply that stick-to-itiveness to your fat loss and health challenges. Specifically, you need to make sure you don't become discouraged after those days when you cheat on the food guidelines of the Nashville Diet.

As I've said before, everybody cheats. But not everybody knows how to handle the situation. Here are some important things for you to know.

You may be innocent. Not every "forbidden" bite qualifies as cheating. In fact, it's very important not to implement every food guideline all at once. And it's just as important not to try to eliminate all problem foods cold turkey. (Though I must say that cold turkey itself is not a problem food—if you take off the skin!) A gradual, step-by-step approach naturally means that you still might be partaking of problem foods several weeks or more after you start the food phase of your program. So, if you eat a chocolate bar, don't be too hard on yourself, especially if you were used to eating one every day before you started making changes. Look at *why* you did it—maybe you went more than five hours without eating, or you hadn't been drinking your water, so you were dehydrated, and so on. Use your setbacks as a learning experience as you gradually change your habits for a lifetime.

Old habits die hard. My clients tend to do their cheating with dairy or sugar, and sometimes alcohol. That makes perfect sense, because these are the addictive toxic foods that many folks have spent their lives craving. It's neither realistic nor advisable to expect anybody to completely remove those old companions from their lives any time soon. So when you cheat, notice the food you cheated with. Is it one of your personal problem foods? Is it a typical craved food for your body type? What was the craving like? What might have led to such a craving? Use your journal to explore these issues. Don't treat this kind of "cheating" as a personal failure. Treat it as the learning experience it is.

If you feel sick afterwards, that's a good sign. As you steadily detox your body, you'll become much more aware of the effects of new toxins. What's more, you'll become unable to indulge in your toxic foods the way you used to. Once upon a time, you may have eaten a pound of bacon for breakfast four days a week, oblivious to the damage being done by all that saturated fat, salt, and cured, processed meat. Now, months later, you cheated on your food guidelines and went for a few slices of bacon at the brunch buffet table—and you feel terrible. Congratulations! You've cleansed your body to the point where it won't tolerate a level of toxicity that was once a drop in the bucket for you.

That little bout of cheating demonstrated the progress you made, and now you're much less likely to even want bacon in the future. It's much like an ex-smoker who tries a puff after five years and gags in disgust. Or it's like my chocolate transformation. I used to be able to eat an entire pan of brownies. Now I won't touch even one. It's not willpower. It's not lack of opportunity. It's because even the smell is nauseating to my cleansed body. It is very similar to an alcoholic going through detox, getting away from alcohol completely for several months then thinking they can drink the same amount they did at the peak of their consumption. This kind of indulgence can be very debilitating not just with alcohol but chocolate or dairy as well.

Each of us literally gets "intoxicated" on different items. It's up to you to determine where your problem areas are and learn to indulge only on a periodic, controlled basis. If you haven't already, you will learn how to ebb and flow your nutrient regimen along with your life to make sure your body doesn't get out of control again. One of my clients is a reformed alcoholic. She says that an extra dose in the afternoon of Hormone Helper and Immune Boosters helps her completely lose all her cravings for alcohol for the first time in her adult life. She went down five sizes in only five months—and her vibrant health glow is unbelievable! So learn about your own system.

There may be a hidden reason for your backsliding. Whenever you backslide on your food program, don't waste time castigating yourself. You're not a bad person for it. Nobody's going to punish you for not minding Dr. Marilyn. Instead, look for the reason. We've already talked about needing time to overcome cravings and food addictions. Look for other reasons as well. Did you skimp on your nutrients? Did you wait more than five hours between meals? Were you exposed to toxins in the last few days? Note these things in your journal. Look for patterns. Take any opportunity to learn about your body and how it reacts to your environment, your habits, and the food you eat. Having your vibrant health is a lifelong research project.

It's what you do in the long run that counts. One misstep, or even a bad week, is not the end of the world. Remember, you're not on some fifteen-day miracle crash diet where every minute counts against an imposed deadline. You don't have a deadline. You're pursuing health for life. So your developing good habits matters much more than your transitory bad spells. Forget about what you did yesterday, and focus on what you're going to do today. Buckle up, renew your determination, and move forward.

A planned "cheat day" is a good idea. After you've completed the switch from processed food to live, low-toxic food, try to get in six weeks of honest, cheat-free eating. This may be the period you do your rotation dieting and/or follow your body-type food plan. Once that's done, it's a good idea to allow for one "cheat day" every two weeks. This serves as a check and balance against recurring cravings, as well as a well-deserved treat for all your good work. On your cheat day, go ahead and eat a problem food if you want one. See if you can enjoy a piece of pie (which has refined flour and probably hydrogenated fat, as well as sugar) or some crackers and cheese *without craving it*. Note how you feel the next day—it probably won't be all that good. Enter that in your journal. And be sure to go right back to your good eating habits the next day and cheat no more for two weeks.

An even better way to incorporate your cheat day is to implement it as you follow the recommended diet for your body imbalance. Simply take food from your "0 percent" category (foods you will normally avoid completely) and swap them for foods in your "80 percent" category. For example, I'm a thyroidian, so I crave chocolate, sweets, and caffeine (or at least I used to). So a chocolate bar would have all three of those things, but, honestly, I could never eat one, even on a cheat day. So I'll pull out some other "cheat" foods from my "0 percent" category, and eat things like cereal with bananas, toast, a sandwich, some kind of casserole dish, and a piece of cake.

I'M PASSING YOU THE BATON

When I was about twelve years old, my astute mother realized I needed something constructive to do with my time, so she enrolled me in baton-twirling classes, of all things. And just three years later I was a true "Texas Twirler" —and state champion. But it took endless hours of practice, especially for the "time toss," in which the baton is tossed up in a small circle, caught, and immediately tossed up again. It took me a full week and hundreds of drops before I could catch that baton just once after tossing it up. Once I mastered that, I decided to go for ten catches in a row. If I got to nine in a row and dropped the tenth, I'd start over.

Over the next month I must have dropped and picked up that baton a thousand times. Suffice it to say I didn't get to be state champion by walking away for the day just because of one drop.I learned from what I had done wrong and tried again. Eventually I conquered the time toss. I had stuck with it long enough to make it a habit. What was once a challenge was now a routine. It was easy.

Three years later, however, during my routine at the state championships, guess what—I dropped the baton during the time toss. But you know what? I won anyway. I picked that baton back up, got right back into the routine, and finished a winning performance.

I was able to recover after my blunder because I knew I didn't have to go back to square one after that drop. The payoff from those three years of dedication and practice was still with me and always would be. Not even the worse setback imaginable—a drop at the state championships!— could erase the advantage I'd accumulated from never giving up.

And to this day, I never give up. I may get discouraged. I may regret something I've done. But I never, ever let it deter me from my chosen path. I acknowledge a mistake, see what I can learn from it, and go forward. I can do this because I *decided* to develop good habits—in baton twirling, in matters of health, and in life. Once those habits stick, abandoning them is simply not an option. Do I want to go back to being fat, sick, and bedridden? I don't *think* so. I refuse. Anytime I get off track, I just set my jaw for the rest of the day. And I've learned how to get back on the right track quicker and quicker.

You are just as capable of developing the good health and eating habits outlined in this book. What's more, you and I have an advantage that most people don't. We know a program to follow that helps us achieve our goals. We've discovered a path from fat to lean that emphasizes what matters most: vibrant health. It's so much easier to keep moving ahead when you know you're moving in the right direction. The Nashville Diet was mine. Now it's yours. I've given it to you with full confidence that you'll use it to achieve the success you deserve. I pray God speed for each of you.

THE NASHVILLE DIET STEP-BY-STEP:

twelve weeks to a new you

I recently taught a course on the Nashville Diet and vibrant health to a bright and eager gathering of people from all walks of life who were searching for answers to their health and weight problems.

I was especially impressed by a noticeably overweight man in his mid-sixties who was clearly struggling with a number of health problems and too many prescription medications. He faithfully attended all the classes, took copious notes, and asked all the right questions. He was a joy to teach.

After the sessions, I helped the attendees implement nutrient programs and eating plans for shedding fat and restoring health. But my "star student" —the one who had been so attentive—thanked me profusely for all I'd taught him and then simply left. He made no effort to put his learning to use. He bought no nutrients. He started no program. He was now smarter, but no healthier.

Knowledge is the beginning of wisdom. And true wisdom is knowledge applied. In other words, learning is necessary, but without action it's meaningless. Please don't end up like my star student who learned much but did nothing. You have acquired the knowledge you need to turn your life around. It's time to apply it.

True, there are lots of changes for you to implement as you follow the Nashville Diet. It's quite a challenge. But it's not an overwhelming task if you take things one at a time. Swallow that first nutrient supplement and you've taken the biggest step. Thousands before you have done it with astonishing success. Now it's your turn.

GET GOING AND KEEP GOING

I want to give you two gifts before I leave you on your own to seek and find your vibrant health. One is what I call the Vibrant Health Points System. It's almost like a daily game in which you reward yourself for good, healthy behavior, but you also have to deduct points for those naughty little lapses that impede your progress. It's a very effective way to monitor how you're doing, and to motivate you to do better.

The other tool I'll leave you with is a week-by-week checklist that will guide you through your Nashville Diet program. Use this chart to help you plan and time your implementation of all the strategies you've learned—phasing in your maximum nutrient doses, practicing detox techniques, replacing toxic foods with live foods, starting a light exercise program, drinking plenty of water, and so on.

I suggest you make enough copies of the Vibrant Health Points chart to use daily for twelve weeks, making a copy for each day. I'd put those copies in a three-ring loose-leaf binder, along with your twelve-week checklist and your weekly Vibrant Health Index questionnaires. How you organize this binder is up to you, but you'll find it useful to have all of these things in one, easy-to-access place. You can also include a section in that binder for your daily journal entries, if you like.

THE VIBRANT HEALTH POINTS SYSTEM:
KEEPING TRACK OF YOUR PROGRESS

In Chapter Four, you were introduced to the concept of the Vibrant Health Index, which gives you an idea of how your overall health is responding to your ongoing efforts. The Vibrant Health Points System, how-ever, will tell you what everybody who follows the Nashville Diet always wants to know: "How'd I do today?" and "How do I raise my VHI score?" The VHI tells you how you *are doing*. The daily Vibrant Health Points System shows *what you are doing* that is making you respond.

The Vibrant Health Points System uses an easy-to-follow chart (see Appendix B on p. 259) that divides your health-building efforts toward fat-to-lean into seven categories. The left side of the chart is dedicated to the positive things you can do in each category. The right side deals with the negative aspects. If you exercise for twenty minutes, that's positive. If you skip a meal, that's negative. The chart works by keeping score of the never-ending battle between good and evil; that is, between your health-pro-moting "good" actions and your health-undermining "bad" actions. It does this by having you score a certain amount of points for each good action, and a certain amount of points for each bad action. The positive points, entered on the left side of the chart, are Health-Building Points (HBPs); the negative points are Toxic/Chemicals Points (TCPs). At the end of the day, you simply add up the points on each side. Then you subtract the negative point total (TCPs) from the positive point total (HBPs) to get your score for the day. That score can be as high as the 120s.

But don't be surprised (or overly concerned) if your score's a negative number, meaning you accumulated more negative TCPs that day than positive HBPs. That's nothing to be ashamed of in the early stages of your program. In fact, it makes perfect sense. If you were doing everything right each day, you'd probably already have your vibrant health. What you want, of course, is to see those scores start trending toward the positive side as you acquire more of the good habits you've learned. Most people find that as soon as their daily Vibrant Health Points consistently are in the 80s and above, their VHI will begin rising up fairly rapidly.

KEEPING SCORE

Take a glance at the Vibrant Health Points System charts in Appendix B so you get an idea of how the categories break down. Then read on to learn what numbers to put in the boxes based on your health behavior each day. We'll run down the score-keeping details category by category.

Nutrition

Health-Building Points. The only entry on the HBP side in the nutrition category is for your nutraplenishing. You get 2 points for every minimum dose of every group of recommended nutrients that you take. For example, if you take one dose of all your Immune Boosters, give yourself 2 points. If you've moved up to two doses of Immune Boosters daily, give yourself 4 points for that. If you're at a stage where you're taking two or more doses of all five nutrient groups, your HBP score for this entry may soar into the 20s or even the 30s.

Toxic/Chemicals Points. The negative side of the nutrition equation is where you'll deduct points for prescription medicines, over-the-counter medications, and chemical (as opposed to natural) vitamins. Antidepressants, hormone replacement medications, birth control, ibuprofen, and Tylenol all fall into this category. Take 2 points off for each typical dosage of any of those things you take on a given day, but do not skip a prescribed medication just to score points. Keep taking your medications until your doctor says you can stop.

Food

Health-Building Points. For each of the three meals you eat in a day; give yourself 15 points just for eating it. Use the space in the chart for each meal to write down what you ate, but the content doesn't affect your HBP. This needs to be a "real" meal, not a candy bar and a soft drink. If you ate the meal, you get 15 points. For the "water" entry below the three meals, give yourself 1 point for every 10 ounces of approved distilled water you drank that day, and ½ point for every 10 ounces of tap water that you drank.

Toxic/Chemicals Points. Here's where you lose points for eating the wrong foods during those 15-point meals. And you'll probably lose plenty of points until you really start making significant progress in implementing the eating guidelines and strategies given in Chapters Ten and Eleven. For each meal, consider the following for your TCPs:

- ☐ 4 points for each food that is not organic.
- ☐ 3 points for each food that is highly processed (fast food included).
- ☐ 4 points for each fried food in that meal.
- ☐ 4 points for any food you eat that contains more than three nonfood chemicals, or if it includes caffeine or sugar.
- ☐ 10 points if you skipped that meal.
- ☐ 5 points if you ate less than four hours or more than five hours since your last meal. Deduct 5 points if you go longer than 2 hours without eating after you get up in the morning.
- ☐ 5 points for each snack you had before that meal.
- ☐ 5 points for not drinking any water for the day. 1 additional point for every 12 ounces of soft drink, coffee, or nonherbal tea (most fruit teas are not true herbal teas) you consumed during the day.

You can readily see how the "bad" food points can add up quickly to give you a negative overall food score. A worst-case scenario might be skipping a meal and having a chocolate candy bar and a cola instead. You'll have to dock yourself 10 points for the skipped meal (in addition to getting 0 HBPs for that meal instead of 15), 10 points for the snacks (5 for the candy bar and 5 for the coke), 8 points for the chemicals/caffeine/sugar in both of them, 8 points for two nonorganic foods, 6 points for two highly processed foods. That's a negative 42 points right there, and it could be more if you ate that candy bar and drank that soft drink before four hours had passed since your last meal. Just one slip like that can put you hopelessly in the hole for the entire day! One more thing: If that cola you drank was 24 ounces—a medium-size drink (we're not talking "Big Gulp")—you have to multipy your TCP numbers times 3!!

Many people think, "Oh, I'll cheat but then I'll work it off (or I'll skip a meal and eat this instead)." If that's you, you're in for a big surprise! If you drink a medium Coke and eat a candy bar (Almond Joy or a bag of Reese's Pieces) or a sweet roll (Honey Bun), you'll be consuming almost 500 calories.

Guess how much exercise it will take to "work it off"? Not walking, not jogging but in a dead run the likes of which would cause most American adults over the age of twenty-five to fall over dead after two blocks. Running at that pace—five miles per hour—it would take one full hour to "run it off." One hour!!

STOP IT, AMERICA!!!

Exercise
Health-Building Points. Give yourself 10 HBPs if you exercise between twenty and forty-five minutes that day.

Toxic/Chemicals Points. Give yourself 5 TCPs if you fail to exercise that day (even if it's your rest day).

Exposure to Sun
I haven't talked much about sun exposure. As is well publicized, overexposure can be dangerous. But a moderate amount of indirect sun exposure is beneficial for efficient absorption of vitamins D and C. It can also help your body produce serotonin. Being out in the sun before 9 A.M. each day can reset your body clock and help you sleep better at night. Combining some indirect sun with outdoor exercise or a walk would be ideal.

Health-Building Points. Give yourself 4 points for ten to forty minutes of indirect sun exposure.

Toxic/Chemicals Points. Deduct 2 TCPs if you get no sun at all that day or if you get more than forty minutes of exposure.

Toxic Elimination

Health-Building Points. After you've worked your way up to and then completed your detox regimen, continuing to perform two of the treatments will get you HBPs. Score 2 positive points for doing a lymphatic massage and 2 positive points for doing a dry skin brush. Give yourself 2 HBPs for each healthy bowel movement you have. (A healthy bowel movement has a soft stool that's easily and naturally passed.)

   Toxic/Chemicals Points. There is no TCP penalty for not doing a lymphatic massage or a dry skin brush on any one day. Instead, use the space under Toxic/Chemicals to note any new or unusual negative feelings on that day. There will be no points off for those feelings, however. Score 5 TCPs if you have less than one healthy bowel movement.

Toxic Exposure

Health-Building Points. Give yourself 4 positive points for a day marked by healthy stress. Healthy stress describes a challenging situation that you feel competent to cope with and that you handle successfully with a sense of accomplishment. Use the rest of the space to note any new or unusual positive feelings that arose that day, Sorry, no points here—just observation.

   Toxic/Chemicals Points. Score 10 points for a day marked by negative stress. Negative stress is a troublesome situation or encounter that you find difficult to manage and that gives you a churning, overwhelmed feeling. Deduct 10 to 15 TCPs for any incidence of ongoing toxic exposure in your home, work space, or elsewhere. Score 50 TCPs if you were unfortunate enough to be subjected to a one-time environmental exposure—like finding yourself in a mold-ridden building while visiting.

Sleep

Health-Building Points. Because vibrant health depends on the rebuilding and repair that adequate sleep offers, give yourself 4 HBPs for getting six to ten hours of sleep.

Toxic/Chemicals Points. Deduct 5 TCPs if you sleep fewer than six hours or 5 TCPs if you sleep more than ten hours, since this is usually an indication of some toxicity.

LEARNING FROM YOUR VIBRANT HEALTH POINTS

The Vibrant Health Points System is an excellent learning tool. Some beginners find that getting a daily "grade" can be enlightening and motivating; others feel they have enough to do without filling out a points chart every day. Some veteran Nashville Dieters appreciate the clear picture they get from the chart and the score it gives; others simply don't need a number to tell them how they're doing. They're familiar enough with all the program components and their own habits to keep a virtual running tally in their heads. I encourage beginners to use the chart and point system, however. I've found that it really helps to have some kind of objective evaluation of your program compliance. Otherwise, to put it bluntly, it's too easy to fool yourself into thinking your health habits are better than they are. If you want to wait a week or two before charting yourself with the points system, that's fine. But get to it earlier rather than later. I've always found the points chart useful when clients comment, "I'm doing *everything* and still not losing weight." If they keep the chart for even one week, there is so much light shed that usually we can get them moving in the desired direction.

The points system will help you in other ways besides just keeping score:

It's a daily reminder. The system is designed to remind you daily of all the specific things you need to do or not do to get your VHI up and your weight down.

It points out trouble spots. It alerts you to certain areas that cause you the most trouble. For example, if you review your charts for the last two weeks and see that you're consistently losing points for eating nonorganic, you're reminded of what you need to work on. You may not have realized that your VHI progress has been stalled because you're still getting too many chemicals in your otherwise admirable diet.

It's a visual reminder. The chart offers a visual reminder that the past is past and that each day begins with a new slate. That big number 50 on the TCP side for replacing a meal with a cola and candy bar yesterday turns back to a 0 the next morning, inspiring you to move on and do well, rather than wallow in remorse for your lapse.

It suggests strategies. The chart can suggest strategies for compensating for unavoidable "bad" behavior by emphasizing the good things available for you. For example, you can see that your health is suffering each day from an ongoing environmental toxic exposure in your home because the mold remediation guys can't schedule you in for another month. That's something you can't do much about for a while. But a glance over at the HBP side might suggest that you can compensate somewhat by upping your water and nutrient intake and doing lemon pushes until they can get there.

It shows your behavior patterns. You can spot behavior patterns and variations by studying your points charts. Perhaps you usually have more cravings in the afternoon than any other time. Or you often skip meals on certain days when your schedule is busier. Or you tend to miss your nutrient doses on weekends. The charts can help you spot those trends and suggest ways to correct the problems.

It's yours alone. Mainly, though, the chart (like your journal and the pace with which you implement the Nashville Diet) is something that belongs to you and you alone. It's *your* personal tool. It reflects only *your* habits, *your* strengths, and *your* weaknesses. That's one of the fundamental realities of this program and everything else you do to improve yourself as a person. It's your body, your health, your life. What happens with them is ultimately your choice. I've shown you the path from fat to lean. It's up to you to follow it. I know that you can and you will. And I promise you that you'll be grateful the rest of your life that you did.

YOUR NASHVILLE DIET WEEK-BY-WEEK GUIDE AND CHECKLIST

Most followers of the Nashville Diet experience significant progress within twelve weeks: smaller clothing sizes, more energy, the vibrant health glow, weight loss, a balanced, happier disposition, and elevated self-esteem. But everybody progresses at their own pace, so the week-by-week checklist I've prepared for you has to be considered a *typical* plan of action, not the *only* plan of action. Use it as a guide, not a strict list of instructions. Many times, your VHI or other factors simply won't allow you to complete every recommended action in a given week. Yet you'll be able to complete others. Check off each action you do carry out. At the end of the week, circle the area to the left of each action you chose not to complete. That will remind you to come back to that after you move forward.

Always refer to the chapter or chapters where each action was presented before carrying it out. It's more important to do things right than to do them right away. The wording of the actions on this checklist is necessarily brief. You'll often need more information about what to do, and I certainly don't expect you to remember every detail of what you've already read. When you make that first check mark during Week One, you've started on a magnificent journey that will transform you into the lean and energetic lover of life that you really are.

Relax, take it slow, and enjoy yourself!

WEEK ONE

__Vow to do what it takes to get healthy and lean.

__Weigh yourself and then put the scale away for a month. If a tape measure is available, measure chest, waist, hips, thighs, and upper arms. (If no tape measure is available do NOT let this keep you from starting.) Another option is to have your fat percentage or your body mass index taken at a local gym.

__Take your first Vibrant Health Index (VHI) (see Chapter Four).

__Begin journaling.

—Determine which nutrients you need to buy, based on your VHI.

—Buy the nutrients.

—Begin taking Immune Boosters at the minimum level for your VHI.

—Add Fregetables on the third day.

—Add Hormone Helpers on the fifth day.

—Make a point to drink a 4-ounce glass of clean water in the morning, one at mid-day and one in the afternoon, each day.

WEEK TWO

—Take your VHI on your VHI day (Sunday or Monday is best; be consistent).

—Continue taking your nutrients daily.

—Phase in Masters of Metabolism if your VHI is 70 + (be sure to "rotate"; see Chapter Four).

—Begin raising some nutrient-group dosages if it's time to (see Chapter Four).

—Buy a water bottle and drink at least 32 ounces each day (that's eight 4-ounce glasses).

—Continue journaling.

WEEK THREE

—Take your VHI on your VHI day.

—If your VHI is over 70, phase in Detox Delights.

—Make appropriate adjustments of your nutrient doses if it's time to do so.

—Up your water intake to 48 ounces a day (that's twelve 4-ounce glasses, or two 32-ounce bottles).

—List the problem foods you need to eliminate (see Chapters Nine and Ten).

—Start making sure you allow four hours between meals, but no more than five.

—Make it a point to get a few minutes of sun every day, if possible.

—Keep journaling.

—Inventory your nutrients and buy what you need in advance for the second month.

Week Four

—Take your VHI on your VHI day.

—All your nutrient groups should be at maximum dosage, if your VHI allows.

—Begin phasing in the Detox Delights if your VHI is 70 + .

—Eliminate two problem foods from your diet and replace them with live food.

—Spend some time in a good health food store, looking at labels and food choices.

—Up your water intake to 64 ounces a day (that's 16 4-ounce glasses, or two 32-ounce bottles).

—Start taking a walk every day, even if it's only down the block.

—Shop for a mini-trampoline for future rebound exercise.

—Keep journaling.

Week Five

—Congratulate yourself for finishing the first and hardest one-month phase of your Nashville Diet journey!

—Weigh yourself and then put the scale away for a month. If a tape measure is available, measure chest, waist, hips, thighs, and upper arms. (If no tape measure is available, do NOT let this keep you from starting.) Another option is to have your fat percentage or your body mass index taken at a local gym.

—Take your VHI on your VHI day.

—Journal at least three times this week on your daily Vibrant Health Points Chart.

—Keep taking all your nutrients at the top dosage your VHI allows.

—Up your water intake to 88 ounces a day.

—Eliminate more problem foods from your diet, shifting to a majority of live food.

—On Monday, begin daily lymphatic massages and diaphragmatic breathing (see Chapter Six).

—On Tuesday, do a lemon push and a dry skin brush (see Chapter Six).

__On Wednesday through Saturday, try your hand at the very simple tai chi exercises described in Chapter Six. Practice one stage a day for five to ten minutes.

__On the weekend, get into some beginning rebounding on your mini-trampoline (see Chapter Six).

__Stretch your daily walk time to at least ten minutes if you can. Try one twenty-minute walk on the weekend if you're up to it.

__Keep journaling.

WEEK SIX

__Take your VHI on your VHI day.

__Keep taking all your nutrients faithfully at the top dosage your VHI allows.

__Journal every day this week on your daily VHP chart.

__If you can increase your water intake beyond 88 ounces a day, start this week. (Your top goal is 128 ounces a day, but don't push it. You're fine at 88 for now.)

__Eliminate the remaining "bad" foods from your diet list. Try to make this the week that live food and the other guidelines in Chapter Ten completely replace processed and other toxic food.

__Start phasing in organic versions of all your food categories.

__On Monday, try the hot-and-cold shower hydrotherapy treatment (see Chapter Six).

__This week, if you feel ready and your VHI is at least 65, start your seven-treatment detox regimen, as described in Chapter Six. Follow it daily for three weeks, and then only do individual treatments as needed. After the regimen, you can continue tai chi if you wish, and you have the option of adapting the rebounding as your cardiovascular exercise.

__Stretch your daily walk time to at least twenty minutes if you can. Try one thirty-minute walk on the weekend if you're up to it. For added benefit, get your walking in while there's indirect (midmorning or midafternoon) sun.

__Keep journaling.

WEEK SEVEN

—Take your VHI on your VHI day.

—Keep taking all your nutrients faithfully at the top dosage your VHI allows.

—Inventory your nutrients and purchase what you'll need for the third month.

—Journal every day this week on your DVHP chart.

—Continue with the second week of your three-week detox regimen, if you started last week. If you didn't, you may start it this week if you can.

—On Monday, begin the environmental cleanup and mold inspection of your home, as outlined in Chapter Seven. Start with your bedroom and do one room each day.

—Spend some more time in a local health food store, seeking new healthy alternatives.

—Strive to get as close as you can to 100 percent live food, 100 percent organic food, and 0 percent "problem" food.

—Keep drinking at least 88 ounces of water a day.

—Keep journaling.

WEEK EIGHT

—Take your VHI on your VHI day.

—Keep taking all your nutrients faithfully at the top dosage your VHI allows.

—Journal every day this week on your DVHP chart.

—Complete the third week of your three-week detox regimen.

—Make an effort to add at least one "new" healthy food to your diet each day, starting with the recommendations in Chapter Ten.

—Continue with your in-house environmental cleanup if you didn't finish last week.

—Inventory your household cleaning and personal hygiene products. Replace any two toxic products with a healthier alternative (see Chapter Seven). Spend time at a local health food store looking at natural/organic personal hygiene and cleaning products.

Week Nine

—Congratulate yourself on a successful second month on the Nashville Diet.

—Pull out your scale, weigh yourself, and then put the scale away again.

—Take your VHI on your VHI day.

—Journal every day this week on your DVHP chart.

—Keep taking all your nutrients faithfully at the top dosage your VHI allows.

—Replace two more toxic household cleaning or personal hygiene products with healthy alternatives this week, if possible.

—Keep drinking at least 88 ounces of water a day.

—Work at least fifteen minutes per day on environmental cleanup, either in your home or your place of work, or by adjusting your outdoor routine to avoid toxicity.

—On Monday, begin your cardiovascular exercise program. If you're already walking five times a week, you're ahead of the game. That's also true if you decided to continue rebounding as an aerobic exercise. In any case, start working up to a half hour of cardio training five times a week.

—If you've finished your three-week detox regimen, continue to do your diaphragmatic breathing and lymph massage daily. Do the other techniques occasionally or as needed.

—Keep journaling.

Week Ten

—Take your VHI on your VHI day.

—Journal every day this week on your DVHP chart.

—Keep taking all your nutrients faithfully at the top dosage your VHI allows.

—Keep drinking at least 88 ounces of water a day.

—Look for more opportunities to replace toxic household cleaning or personal hygiene products with healthy alternatives.

—On Tuesday or later in the week, begin your twice-a-week strength-training program, as outlined in Chapter Eight.

—If you've eliminated almost all problem foods in favor of almost all good, healthy, live food that's mostly organic for three weeks now, start rotation dieting this week. See Chapter Eleven for instructions. Continue until you reach your goal weight and/or your VHI gets to the 90s and consistently stays there.

—Continue your environmental cleanup work for fifteen minutes a day.

—Continue your twice-weekly strength-training and your five-times-a-week cardio work. Increase your cardio workout time by ten minutes a day if it's not already up to thirty minutes a day.

—Keep journaling.

WEEK ELEVEN

—Take your VHI on your VHI day.

—Keep taking all your nutrients faithfully at the top dosage your VHI allows.

—Take inventory of your nutrients and buy what you need for the fourth month.

—Keep drinking at least 88 ounces of water a day.

—Increase your strength training to three days a week.

—Continue your rotation dieting, lowering the low-calorie day calorie count by 25 percent if you're working your way down to the minimum.

—Continue vigilant environmental cleanup at regular intervals. If you find it useful, continue with the fifteen-minute daily cleanup work.

—Add your Body Type Food Program (see Chapter Twelve).

—Journal every day this week on your DVHP chart. Pay particular attention to eating and journaling on your Body Type Food Program.

WEEK TWELVE

—Take your VHI on your VHI day.

—Keep taking all your nutrients faithfully at the top dosage your VHI allows.

—Keep drinking at least 88 ounces of water a day.

—Continue your rotation dieting, lowering the low-calorie day calorie count by 25 percent if you're working your way down to the minimum. Consider implementing the body type diet plan to move your VHI higher (see Chapter Eleven). You may start the Body Type dieting as early as Week Nine (and simultaneously with rotation dieting) if you're not overwhelmed by too much to do.

—Keep journaling at least three days a week.

BEYOND WEEK TWELVE

—Continue to take your VHI once a week until it levels off in the 90s and you reach your ideal body weight.

—Weigh yourself once a month.

—When you finish your rotation dieting, you will notice a clear VHI improvement and some welcome fat loss at that point. And you'll be feeling much better. If not, troubleshoot for factors that may be impeding your progress (see Chapter Twelve) and start keeping your DVHPs for a week to see if you can find the problem.

—You may plan for a "cheat day" every other week (see Chapter Twelve).

—Once you have reached your goal of VHI in the 90s and your ideal weight, you can cut back to doing your VHI monthly instead of weekly.

—At the same time you calculate your monthly VHI, inventory your stock and re-order or adjust your nutrients.

—If your monthly VHI ever drops more than 2 points, your clothes feel a little snug, or your cravings seem to be edging back in, then immediately add an additional dose of nutrients each day, track your DVHPs for a week, and then take your VHI again. Keep doing this until your VHI drops back down or your weight stops edging up.

YOUR LEAN AND HEALTHY FUTURE STARTS NOW!

You've done it! You've taken the time to become aware of a totally new approach to fat loss. You're ready to use the Nashville Diet to move from fat to lean, and to feel better than you ever have in your life.

But before you do anything else, congratulate yourself for breaking free of the get-thin-quick myth. That alone is a remarkable achievement that puts you in a very elite class indeed. Then continue to congratulate yourself every step of the way along your journey from fat to lean. By seeking weight loss via improving your internal health, you've assured your own success.

I insisted at the very beginning of our journey together that there is hope for you to overcome your weight and health issues and live an active, happy, and fulfilling life. Remember? Well, you've uncovered through your diligent reading the source of that hope. I think you can see now that the hope I referred to wasn't some vague sense of optimism. Instead, it's a real, concrete hope that comes straight from the specific strategies that make up the Nashville Diet.

Never give up that hope as you face the challenges and rewards that lie ahead. Remember that I'm living proof that success is possible. Every detail of the Nashville Diet grew out of my own experiences, my own suffering, my own determination to get healthy and lean. I got there, and I've given you this program so you'll get there too. Vibrant health is a blessing you deserve.

vibrant health index questionnaire

on the following pages you'll find the Vibrant Health Index questionnaire, which you first read about in Chapter Four. The VHI will help get you successfully on the road from fat to lean. But please don't write your answers down in this book. It's best if you make several photocopies of this questionnaire: You'll be taking your "Vibrant Health" pulse many times over the next several days, weeks, and months as you follow your Nashville Diet program.

For the sake of convenience, you can go to the www.nashvillediet. com Web site and take the index online, where it will calculate your Vibrant Health Index and the amount of each nutrient you'll need to take for your current VHI.

For you math whizzes out there, or if you don't have access to a computer, the old-fashioned way will work, too: Make 12 copies of the VHI, since you will be taking the VHI every week, optimally on the same night of the week for 12 weeks. To score, simply add your score from each of the 32 questions, divide the total by two and subtract that number from 100; this is your individual VHI.

VIBRANT HEALTH INDEX

Unless otherwise indicated, rate your level of health TODAY on a scale from 0–5 ("5" being the most severe or intense, and "0" being the least or no problem at all). Write your score in the space to the right. If it says "score × 2," double your choice.

1. How do you feel today? score ☐

   "UNDER THE BED" 5 · 4 · 3 · 2 · 1 · 0 "TOP OF THE WORLD"

2. Describe your energy level. score × 2 ☐

   CHRONIC FATIGUE 5 · 4 · 3 · 2 · 1 · 0 FULL OF ENERGY

3. Describe your headaches.

   For each type of headache, evaluate the amount of pain and frequency, "5" being at least one or two headaches per week that interfere with your normal activity, and "0" being no more than one a year.

   migraines 5 · 4 · 3 · 2 · 1 · 0 score ☐
   sinus 5 · 4 · 3 · 2 · 1 · 0 score ☐
   other 5 · 4 · 3 · 2 · 1 · 0 score ☐

4. Assess the health of your joints. score ☐

   A "5" means severe arthritis or other joint pain, requiring prescription medication.

   SEVERE 5 · 4 · 3 · 2 · 1 · 0 PAIN-FREE JOINTS

5. Do you have chronic muscle pain? score ☐

   Consider chronic pain only, not the occasional "sore muscle." Don't include muscle spasms or pain related to back strain, back injury, or other muscle pain relating to trauma. A "5" would indicate you suffer from severe, chronic muscle pain, that you're taking prescription medication for muscle pain at least twice a week, or that you've been diagnosed with fibromyalgia. A "0" means you're free of any chronic muscle pain.

   SEVERE 5 · 4 · 3 · 2 · 1 · 0 PAIN-FREE

6. Describe your menstrual symptoms. score ☐

   Consider pain, PMS, mood swings, and chocolate or other food cravings related to menstruation. "0" means you're symptom-free before, during, and after menstruation. If any of your symptoms are severe, score "5".

   SEVERE 5 · 4 · 3 · 2 · 1 · 0 PAIN-FREE

7. Do you have menopausal symptoms? score ☐

   This question applies to postmenopausal women and women who have had their ovaries removed. Grade the severity of hot flashes, dramatic mood swings, crying, etc.

   SEVERE SYMPTOMS 5 · 4 · 3 · 2 · 1 · 0 NO SYMPTOMS

8. How's your sex drive? score ☐

   ZERO INTEREST 5 · 4 · 3 · 2 · 1 · 0 HIGH DESIRE, SATISFACTION

9. How well do you manage stress? score ☐

   EASILY OVERWHELMED 5 · 4 · 3 · 2 · 1 · 0 COPE WELL

10. How susceptible are you to colds, other viral infections? score ☐

   MORE THAN 5 A YEAR 5 · 4 · 3 · 2 · 1 · 0 ONE EVERY FEW YEARS

1 1. How well do you concentrate?   score ☐

ALWAYS AWAKE, ALERT   5 · 4 · 3 · 2 · 1 · O   IN A FOG MOST OF THE TIME

1 2. How's your memory?   score ☐

FREQUENTLY FORGETFUL 5 · 4 · 3 · 2 · 1 · O RARELY FORGET ANYTHING IMPORTANT

1 3. Are you depressed?   score ☐

ON MEDICATION   5 · 4 · 3 · 2 · 1 · O   RARELY FEEL DOWN FOR LONG

1 4. Evaluate your sleep habits.   score ☐

If you have difficulty falling asleep more than three nights per week, or wake up twice
or more a night for no apparent reason, score "5". "O" means you almost always fall
asleep easily and sleep soundly.

FREQUENT DIFFICULTY   5 · 4 · 3 · 2 · 1 · O   SOUND SLEEPER

1 5. Do you have food cravings?   score ☐

DAILY, AND UNCONTROLLABLY 5 · 4 · 3 · 2 · 1 · O RARELY, AND CONTROLLED

1 6. Assess the quality of your bowel movements.   score ☐

"5" means you're almost always either constipated or with diarrhea. "O" is for those
with consistently soft and easily passed stools.

DIFFICULT, INCONSISTENT   5 · 4 · 3 · 2 · 1 · O   SOFT, EASILY PASSED

1 7. Assess the frequency of your bowel movements.   score ☐

LESS THAN ONE A DAY   5 · 4 · 3 · 2 · 1 · O   TWO OR MORE A DAY.

1 8. Do you ever feel bloated?   score ☐

The bloating in question here is not from water retention but from gassiness due to poor
digestion.

SEVERE, VERY FREQUENT   5 · 4 · 3 · 2 · 1 · O   RARE, IF EVER

1 9. Do you suffer from heartburn or indigestion?   score ☐

SEVERE, AFTER MOST MEALS   5 · 4 · 3 · 2 · 1 · O   RARE, IF EVER

20. Is cellulite a problem?   score ☐

IN MORE THAN ONE LARGE AREA   5 · 4 · 3 · 2 · 1 · O   NONE AT ALL

2 1. Do you have allergies or hay fever?   score ☐

Give yourself a "5" if you suffer from allergy symptoms most of the time and haven't
pinned down the cause to one or two things.

FREQUENT SYMPTOMS   5 · 4 · 3 · 2 · 1 · O   NO ALLERGIES OR HAY FEVER

22. Assess your muscle   score ☐

Consider visible muscle, definition, whether you appear firm or "wasted" (regardless of
your weight), and your strength.

VERY POOR   5 · 4 · 3 · 2 · 1 · O   WELL ABOVE AVERAGE

23. Do you have body odor or bad breath?   score ☐

PERSISTENT PROBLEM   5 · 4 · 3 · 2 · 1 · O   RARELY, IF EVER

24. Do you have yeast or fungal infections?   score ☐

Unless you have none ("O") rank your problem by frequency or constancy and symptoms. "5" would mean recurrent or constant infections, accompanied by cravings for
sweets, and chronic achiness and fatigue.

RECURRING, SYMPTOMATIC   5 · 4 · 3 · 2 · 1 · O   RARELY, IF EVER

25. Assess your urinary health.   score ☐

The issue here is whether you have any diagnosed conditions in the urinary tract or problems urinating. A "5" will have been diagnosed with recurrent bladder infections, kidney infection, or severe, chronic urination problems.

SEVERE CONDITION   5 · 4 · 3 · 2 · 1 · 0   NO PROBLEMS

26. Do you smoke?   score ☐

Yes, score "6" · Smoked in the past but no longer do, score "2"
Never smoked, score "0"

27. Do you drink caffeine-containing beverages?   score ☐

That includes coffee, soft drinks, non-herbal tea, and any other drink with caffeine in it. Your score is the number of caffeine-containing drinks you consume per day. If you drink more than five, your score is "5".

28. How overweight are you?   score ☐

Determine (approximately) your ideal weight and the number of pounds you need to lose to get to it.

I'm already at my ideal weight.	0	I need to lose 30 to 44 pounds.	6
I need to lose fewer than 15 pounds.	2	I need to lose 45 to 59 pounds.	8
I need to lose 15-29 pounds.	4	I need to lose 60 or more pounds.	10

29. Do you have pets?   score ☐

Your score is the number of warm-blooded pets you live with. If you have more than five, your score is "5".

30. Do you take any kind of medicine?   score × 2 ☐

Count any kind of medication —prescription, over-the-counter, herbal or homeopathic— that you're taking now. Anything you normally take on an as-needed basis also counts, such as aspirin or an antacid. Your score is the number you take. If you take more than five, your score is "5" (which you'll double to "10").

31. Are you taking any of the following medications?   score × 2 ☐

Check any category of medications for which you take one or more. Your total number of checks is your score (which you'll double). Your maximum score is "10" (doubled to "20")

__High blood pressure medication   __Heart medication
__Water retention medication   __Thyroid disease medication
__Antidepressant   __Diabetes medication
__Glaucoma medication   __MAO inhibitor (monoamine oxidase inhibitor)
__Blood thinner or Coumadin

__Any medication containing ephedrine, pseudoephedrine, or phylopropanolamine.(Includes any allergy medications that contain a decongestant, and all over-the-counter cold medications.)

32. Are you under a doctor's care for any of the following conditions?   score ☐

Your score is the total number checked, up to 10.

__Allergies/Asthma   __Fibromyalgia
__Arthritis   __Glaucoma
__Chronic fatigue syndrome   __Heart disease
__Depression   __Hormone imbalance (of any kind)
__Diabetes

your total VHI index ☐

daily vibrant health points system

on the pages that follow, you'll find two different versions of the Daily Vibrant Health Points System form.

The first chart is the "key" form, and indicates how many Health-Building or Toxic/Chemicals points to assign yourself for each daily activity.

The second chart is a blank form for you to photocopy and fill in daily. Instructions for completing the form are as follows:

1. Assign both Health-Building Points (HBPs) and Toxic/ Chemicals Points (TCPs) to items as instructed in the key chart. Complete all nonshaded areas.
2. Add all HBPs and place the total in the Total Health-Building Points box at the bottom of the chart.
3. Add all TCPs and place the total in the Total Toxic/ Chemicals Points box at the bottom of the chart.
4. Complete the formula given at the bottom of the form-subtract your TCP value from your HBP value-to obtain your total Vibrant Health Points value for the day.

Daily Vibrant Health Points System Key (1)

Day: Date:

Health-Building Points	HBP	Toxic/Chemicals Points	TCP
Nutrition		**Nutrition**	
Approved supplemental nutrients	2 per capsule	Toxic chemicals/pharmaceuticals	2 per capsule or tablet
Food		**Food**	
Time Breakfast	15	Nonorganic	4
(Use this space to record foods eaten.)		Highly processed or fast food	3
		Fried	4
		Contains lists of chemicals, sugar, wheat, dyes, bleaches	4
		Skipped meal	10
		Less than 4 or more than 5 hours since last meal	5
		Snacks (e.g., soft drinks, sweets, pretzels)	5 (per snack)
Time Lunch	15	Nonorganic	4
(Use this space to record foods eaten.)		Highly processed or fast food	3
		Fried	4
		Contains lists of chemicals, sugar, wheat, dyes, bleaches	4
		Skipped meal	10
		Less than 4 or more than 5 hours since last meal	5
		Snacks (e.g., soft drinks, sweets, pretzels)	5 (per snack)
Time Dinner	15	Nonorganic	4
(Use this space to record foods eaten.)		Highly processed or fast food	3
		Fried	4
		Contains lists of chemicals, sugar, wheat, dyes, bleaches	4
		Skipped meal	10
		Less than 4 or more than 5 hours since last meal	5
		Snacks (e.g., soft drinks, sweets, pretzels)	5 (per snack)
Water			
Recommended brands	1 per 10 oz (10 max)	No water	5
Tap water	5 per 10 oz (5 max)	Coffee, tea or soft drinks	1 per 12 oz

DAILY VIBRANT HEALTH POINTS SYSTEM KEY (2)

Day: Date:

HEALTH-BUILDING POINTS	HBP	TOXIC/CHEMICALS POINTS	TCP
Exercise		**Exercise**	
20–40 minutes	10	Less than 20 or more than 45 minutes	2
Exposure to Sun		**Exposure to Sun**	
10–40 minutes	4	No sun exposure	2
Toxic Elimination		**Toxic Elimination**	
Skin brushing	2		
Lymphatic stimulation	2		
Healthy bowel movement each day	2 per bm	Less than one healthy bm per day	5
Toxic Exposure		**Toxic Exposure**	
Healthy stress	4	Nonhealthy stress (see chart)	10
		Environment	
		Home (continual)	15
		Office (continual)	10
		One-time environmental exposure	50
		Continued environmental exposure	30
Sleep		**Sleep**	
6–10 hours per night	4	Less than 6 or more than 10 hours per night	5
Total Health-Building Points	☐	**Total Toxic/Chemicals Points**	☐

Daily Vibrant Health Points System Form (1)

Day: _____   Date: _____

Health-Building Points	HBP		Toxic/Chemicals Points	TCP
Nutrition			**Nutrition**	
Approved supplemental nutrients			Toxic chemicals/pharmaceuticals	
	_____			_____
Food			**Food**	
Time ____ Breakfast	_____		Nonorganic	_____
			Highly processed or fast food	_____
			Fried	_____
			Contains lists of chemicals, sugar, wheat, dyes, bleaches	_____
			Skipped meal	_____
			Less than 4 or more than 5 hours since last meal	_____
			Snacks (e.g., soft drinks, sweets, pretzels)	_____
Time ____ Lunch	_____		Nonorganic	_____
			Highly processed or fast food	_____
			Fried	_____
			Contains lists of chemicals, sugar, wheat, dyes, bleaches	_____
			Skipped meal	_____
			Less than 4 or more than 5 hours since last meal	_____
			Snacks (e.g., soft drinks, sweets, pretzels)	_____
Time ____ Dinner	_____		Nonorganic	_____
			Highly processed or fast food	_____
			Fried	_____
			Contains lists of chemicals, sugar, wheat, dyes, bleaches	_____
			Skipped meal	_____
			Less than 4 or more than 5 hours since last meal	_____
			Snacks (e.g., soft drinks, sweets, pretzels)	_____
Water				
Recommended brands	_____		No water	_____
Tap water	_____		Coffee, tea or soft drinks	_____

Daily Vibrant Health Points System Form (2)

Day: Date:

Health-Building Points	HBP	Toxic/Chemicals Points	TCP
Exercise		**Exercise**	
20–40 minutes	_____	Less than 20 or more than 45 minutes	_____
Exposure to Sun		**Exposure to Sun**	
10–40 minutes	_____	No sun exposure	_____
Toxic Elimination		**Toxic Elimination**	
Skin brushing	_____		
Lymphatic stimulation	_____		
Healthy bowel movement each day	_____	Less than one healthy bm per day	_____
Toxic Exposure		**Toxic Exposure**	
Healthy stress	_____	Nonhealthy stress (see chart)	_____
		Environment	
		Home (continual)	_____
		Office (continual)	_____
		One-time environmental exposure	_____
		Continued environmental exposure	_____
Sleep		**Sleep**	
6–10 hours per night	_____	Less than 6 or more than 10 hours per night	_____
Total Health-Building Points	[ ]	**Total Toxic/Chemicals Points**	[ ]

index